# AUTISTICALLY
## *Yours*

## A PATH TO BECOMING YOUR BEST SELF INSIDE AND OUT

# MissNatasha

# DEDICATION

This book is dedicated to those **especially fantastic individuals.**

**Those** who have ever felt different; not like the others.

**This is the book for you!**

# ACKNOWLEDGEMENT

I'd like to acknowledge the Lord! All the shenanigans I've been brought out of, because of God. Thank you very much, my life is forever lifted and Grace Filled.. Thank you all for supporting an Autistic /ADHD Black Canadian, Caribbean individual like myself,

**You are appreciated**

# TABLE OF CONTENTS

# INTRODUCTION

My intention is that you will leave the pages of this book with a greater appreciation for one Black Canadian Caribbean Woman like myself with unseen disabilities. Good Morning, Good Afternoon, Good Evening and Good Night, MissNatasha here. I am a Mental Wellness Creative and Disability Advocate. I am a mother of two and an auntie to many ;) I am grateful to have the ability to write; to read and to present this Autistically Yours with you all.

I'd like to get started by sharing phrases I live by:

## Create Don't Hate
## and
## You can only be you that's all you can do!

Now let's get started. Call it what you like abilities; disabilities, exceptionalities or differences. Some disabilities you can see and some you cannot but be humble, be respectful and loving when you approach. Instead of making up your own stories, and assumptions about another person. No need for self righteous fronts. Whether it be at work or a brief interaction in the store, most individuals with disabilities seen or unseen are amazing. We have been born to do something great in this world just like you. Autistically Yours was written because there aren't many books by Black Autistic Canadian Carribean women out there, I wanted to use my story and voice. I was tired of not being understood or misunderstood, shooed away or ignored when speaking up for myself or about myself.

Being a black woman with unseen exceptionalities, it was difficult to discern the intentions of another. I live in a society that wants to see me small. Without a voice and no sense of self. So I started to build my table in 2010. That table would fit all of the dreams and aspirations of past; present and future.

This table would seat: Positive thoughts about others, No assumptions. Healthy Habits like, Transparency and Generosity. Inner peace and Honesty would always be welcome. Everyone seated at the table would have the ability to give and receive love. Acceptance and Grace would shine bright in the room. Some people want to keep us small because they don't have the courage to be their best self. Some love to live offended, so that they can bypass accountability.

## Have Difficult Conversations!

I wished that I was around people that cared enough to tell me the truth. But I wasn't so lucky. I had a bunch of people throughout my life lie to my face about all sorts of important and non- important topics. I longed for the feeling of peace; happiness, friendship and normalcy. I didn't know that someone like me could ever attain freedom. Virginia Satir, a Family therapist talks about the five freedoms.

# The Five Freedoms:

1. The freedom to see and hear (perceive) what is here and now, rather than what was, will be or should be.

2. The freedom to think what one thinks, rather than what one should think.

3. The freedom to feel what one feels, rather than what one should feel.

4. The freedom to want what one (desire) and to choose what one wants, rather than one should want

5. The freedom to imagine one's own self- actualization, rather than playing a ridgid role or always playing it safe.

Now think for a moment,  would you be fine with someone telling you that you are not able to think for yourself. Perfectionistic systems measure through critical judgments. Judgment implies your measuring my worth because of something inside you not because of your lack of seeing my worth. This cycle dynamic occurs in some families. Some call it the Scapegoat. The one burdened to bare all of the blame. No one stepping up to the plate to hold any of it. One person can't be the problem! One person can't be the solution either. Conflicts and disagreements are going to occur. But how you deal with turmoil is what sets the tone. I'm sure you would be unhappy most times. Not being able to tap into your own personal power. You wouldn't be able to fully accept yourself, you wouldn't be able to look in the mirror. But I am here to let you know that it is definitely possible for you to live a full life, to your standard not the standard of society. I hope that this book brings you joy and a hopeful spirit after you read it.

What do you think disabilities means? What does seen and unseen disabilities really mean? Google says, An invisible disability can include, but is not limited to: cognitive impairment and brain injury; the autism spectrum; chronic illnesses like multiple sclerosis, chronic fatigue, chronic pain, and fibromyalgia; Deaf and/or hard of hearing; blindness and/or low vision; anxiety, ADHD, CPTSD, and many more. The conversation around disabilities isn't really what I'm here to discuss. But some Caribbean families would rather keep things secret; conceal, don't feel, bury it under the blood of Jesus. But when them skeletons come running out, man do you hear the blame and shame that is thrown around. All of a sudden the silent treatment cames. Everyone has to play along with the Mean girls OR ELSE!!!!!!!! Until somebody in the family passes away and then we start the same thing all over again.

The conversation is around being your most authentic self no matter who, or what stands in your path. Is not taken seriously when it comes to persons with disabilities seen or unseen. I want to discuss why society doesn't accept people with exceptionalities as contributors to society. Just because I choose to talk about my own unseen disabilities doesn't mean I'm looking for sympathy or pity. I'm sure respect and acceptance wouldn't be too much to ask. Shame has a way of showing us where we need fine tuning. Shame lets us know we are limited and finite. Shame allows us to make mistakes once and a while. We musnt use shame as a source of tearing others down. We are supposed to be filling our homes with laughter; healing, hope and courage.  For the most part I've encountered individuals who are ignorant or they believe they are the holders of knowledge. They are perfect and without flaw. I have found beautifully imperfect perfect people to love and that love me.

It's splendid; it's marvelous, it's wicked, it's Bless. People who are doing great things in the world; individuals who took lemons and made lemonade, then shared that lemonade with the world. Flaws and all. People who love the lord and don't just talk about looks or superficial things. I noticed the most disingenuous ones doing that the most. I detest those types of people. Assuming that, that's all you have to offer. That's all you know. Telling you to "just be quiet with all that" when you do bring up topics of interest. Questioning you about other people because that's all they came around you for. Asking you to do their dirty work because they are too chicken shit to do it themselves. I could go on but I'll stop here.

In 2015 I wrote this children's book, Exceptionally You, which highlights some different types of disabilities seen and unseen. All of the disabilities listed in the back of the book represent a real live person with an exceptionality and a personality. Disabilities like Autism or CPTSD (Complex Post Traumatic Stress Disorder). You may not see the physical reasoning behind why a person may act a certain way. I want you and all the world to know that you can only be you, that's all you can do! Touching on the everlasting fact that we all asr Exceptional individuals and don't let anyone tell you different. I included that aspect in the book to start the disability conversation. Promoting the rich wealth of community and connection we can build if we can truly be inclusive. Sometimes we only see the flaw and not the person. By the way we can't pray away Autism, it can't be ignored or hidden. By making someone hide who they are is to kill a person's soul. I happen to be Autistic among other wonderful things. The majority of my life I knew that I was very different. I Loved rocks; Glittery things. Spacing out into imaginary worlds. Complained about tags on my clothing, and the way some fabrics felt. I didn't like stockings, they were too itchy. It took a long time to read and write. I loved Ginger beer and Sorrel at Christmas time. Black Cake with tough icing. I used to go to church with my grandmother. Around Christmas time there would be a bazaar where all of the sisters from the church would bring items to sell. I would make sure I had the biggest ziploc bag I could find in order to get some of the leftover icing from Christmas cakes sold. I'd go to my grandmother to ask her friends for me but Mama would say to go and ask them politely yourself. I was so scared the first time I did it but eventually learned that if I helped and used my words I'd get a nice sized icing sugar haul. My teeth don't thank me now but back then I was in heaven. I grew up eating healthy and staying active so this was okay in my eyes.

I wish I knew about what disabilities really meant, when I was younger. I wish I knew about ADHD, I wish someone told me that after you go through trauma you are supposed to get help and not have to go through hard things alone. Growing up, some didn't understand waking up to the smell of porridge in the morning and hardo bread in the morning. Cereal is for suckers, some West Indian folks would say. My grandmother would make chicken foot soup, I was frightened of it. I would ask Mama to please, please not put any chicken foot in my soup. When I grew up I learned that chicken foot soup is very strengthening to the body. I drove my family mad with all of the things I didn't want to touch; or eat or smell or see. Onions and tomatoes that were sauteed. Those textures drove me up the wall. But with Mama's guidance without Grandma's care. I would have not been able to try new things. I wouldn't be as open to new things as I am if it were not for family and being a bit patient with me. That bit of patience helped me to keep glimmers of hope for the future. I knew there were some people that got me, some who understood how it felt. There are some who may feel sorry for another which breeds curiosity. School made me a happy child and a miserable child too. Some call that Cognitive Dissonance. I wished that I had a twin sister that could have been there with me. I'd do all of the difficult things she couldn't stomach and vice versa. Whatever she wasn't good at I'd do for her so we would be even. I'd obsess over GiJoe and Strawberry Shortcake. They'd tell me I had to pick one or the other but I enjoyed the thrill of Transformers and the cuteness of JEM and the Holograms.

I'd line up my books in a row by color and size. I'd stay in the tub and play for what seemed like hours. Now that I think about it there were loads of signs that indicated that I was different. I'd wondered if my parents saw, If they understood that I was different too. I remember when I would stand  in one place in the school yard. While observing in the school yard I would ignore the underhanded comments like; "You don't know what you're doing, or just leave it".

How do I know what I'm saying is true you ask? It was the way I was introduced to others, talked about behind my back or right in ears reach. A perpetrator laughed and said you think that anyone is going to believe you.  It's the way I'd feel being around family. Hearing some of the comments was deflating and gave me a complex for a long, long time.

I would try my darndest to be like everyone else copying the socially acceptable traits that allow you to be accepted and  liked. But what if the acceptance you're looking for comes in the form of the wrong crowd? What if the crowd is not for you? What if one day you don't recognize the person in the mirror in front of you anymore because of masking yourself soo much. Losing yourself trying to please everyone is exhausting, remember you belong here and you have only to believe.

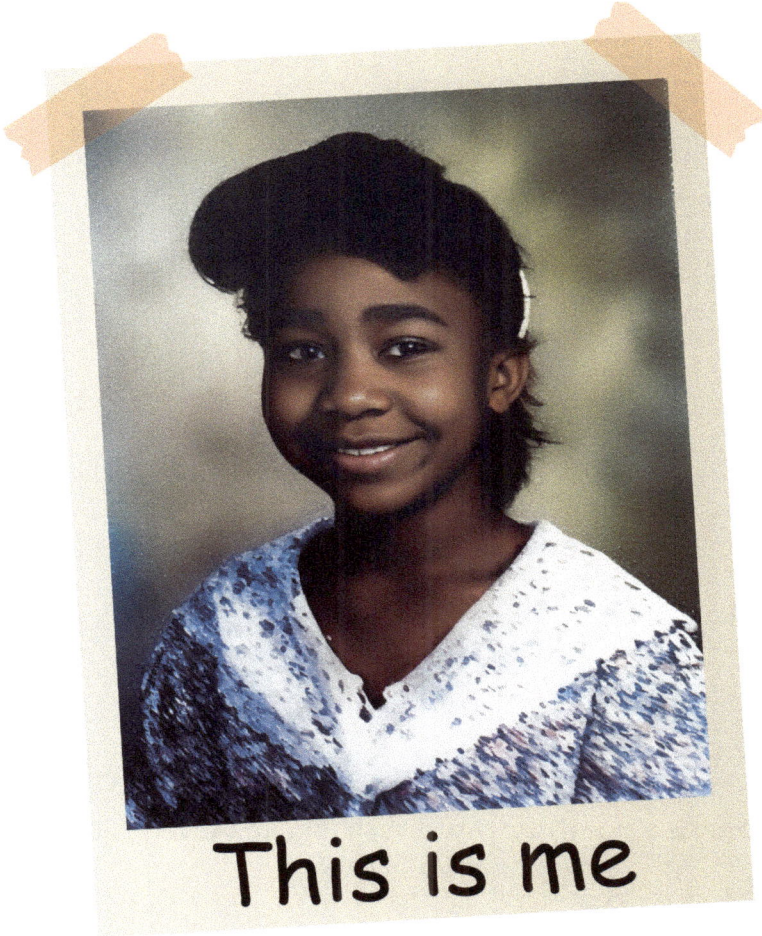

This is me

# Just be you, that's all you can do.

I call myself MissNatasha because most of life I've been incomprehensible, constantly:

Miss Conceived

Miss Educated

Miss Informed

Miss Taken

Miss Understood

Miss Filed

Miss Appropriated

Miss Guided

Miss Interrupted

Miss Construed

Miss Calculated

Miss Managed

Miss filed

I know that I can only be me, that's all I can be.

## MissNatasha 🍓

Don't let others tell you who you are!

# You are you and that's all you can do!

# LET ME BE

## BY: MISSNATASHA

It's okay to show humility when you offend

We are adults we can do the right thing

We can do uncomfortable things

Pick up your feelings and do! Desist from causing problems in your own life by continuing to do old things

Take up your misery and your burdens and cast them away. Free yourself from generational foolishness

Reflect soberly on your doings, your choices, how you affect another

Pivot from negative actions within all aspects of your life

Give others a chance to be successful, without your gatekeeping.

You can give another a chance

# YOU CAN ONLY BE YOU, THAT'S ALL YOU CAN DO!

-MissNatasha

# CHAPTER 1
# JOURNEY TO BECOMING ME

G rowing up, I had mixed emotions about family functions. Activities like BBQs and road trips. I dreaded the thought, because it meant pretending to know what others were talking about during small talk. Knowing what to say. Putting up with the comments my cousins would make;   they'd loved to tease me. Constant reminders of what I couldn't do, what I lacked.  Dogging me out every chance they got, so annoying. I loved learning about who they were and what they did in their daily lives, differing from what I had done. Those interactions carved out some grit into me but did nothing for my self esteem. On the other hand I loved family functions because of sweet treats; the music, seeing familiar faces and of course the delicious Caribbean food. Oxtail; callaloo and crab, cow foot soup, black cake with tough icing. The list of food could go on. I loved the feeling of breaking bread; dumpling or bake with others. Culturally we gathered, told stories of old and prayed together. I Didn't appreciate the chat bout, the clicks, the shame based maneuverings that came along with gatherings. They didn't know me really on a deep personal level, they just presumed to know. It's what happens in a few West Indian households. Blame and shame are the two main players in the game called family.

Made me disgruntled from withdrawn. Finding out things about the world in both negative and positive ways. Having a sense of freedom from reality.

I was presumed to be overactive, over thinker. I accepted that these were the only people that were going to be a part of my world and I did pretty much everything that was asked of me.

As a loner, I oftentimes, entertained myself. I found refuge in music. Patra; Shabba Ranks, Cool Moe Dee, Mary J. Blige and Arrested Development. Repeating and repeating and repeating songs until they jammed up in the tape player. Gatherings were confusing; loud and exciting all wrapped up in one. My moto, consisting of the four F's: food, family, faith, fun. I never really mentioned frustration or facade. I learned about words like frustration; facade and fake later on. When to sit up straight, not to fidget, stand up in Mass, then sit back down, all these different processes and procedures blew my mind, how I managed. Masking, masking made it easier. They said I wasn't agreeable, they said I was too loud or overbearing. Be quiet when in service or when I was around big people. Don't ask questions. Whatever happens in this house stays in this house. It was all so confusing. I'd see one minute we are talking with so and so. The next minute we ain't talking to them again. Back and forth. At the time I had no idea what was different about me.

Usually Caribbean people keep differences to themselves. Not showing weakness. No slipping out of the norm. Keep up appearances! But it is in how we collaborate; how we treat each other in our deep feelings moments and when we are in our egocentric space. I used to think that I was the special one and it was others who needed to catch up. The others knew how to hold eye contact longer or answer quickly without much processing time.

I had gifts and talents too. Growing up I would ask my grandma loads of questions. I wore out my parents ears and needed to know more. I asked where we were from? What was my mother like when she was growing up? I asked how Grandma made her food and what she put into it and why. Such a curious and lonely soul. My Grandma would take us to Mass, when we stayed with her. We would go to the CNE every summer with my cousins. We would go to the movies in Malvern and Scarborough Town Center. Grandma was a force to be reckoned with. I wanted to be like my grandmother's. Confident; independent, they both found love and they both provided the world with acts of service. Both my grandmother's had a couple of children and came to Canada from the Caribbean to provide their families with a better life.

I understood why I was able to learn and adapt in life, God spoke to me on my terms, so I could understand how to maneuver in my own way. Building my resilience and hope in Him. I had to practice, when to keep quiet; practice when to speak up. Practice listening. Being still. I had practiced what I would say and how I would say it for future scenarios. Practice was somewhat exhausting and it made me irritated and upset most of the time. No one was understanding me. I didn't think that I could tell others what was happening to me. I used to think my only friends were going to be my grandmothers, I thought that was cool but when I started big school (elementary) the other children didn't think that having grandma's as friends was fun and they commented that I was weird. I would often question my grandma's about life and how to think or feel about different scenarios. My grandmothers would always refer to the bible and how we are meant to live and behave in the world. Being with my grandparents helped me understand my parents.

My grandmothers helped me to understand more than my little mind would be allowed to process. As some West Indian parents would say, "Stop mining, big people's business."

I couldn't help it. If the children are running me and saying get lost and the big people. What would you have me do? Sit somewhat quietly and observe. Accidently comment or ask a question. I learned a lot. There wasn't much that I had in common with the other children around me so I'd spend time where the older people were. Gaining insights about a life I had not lived as yet. I didn't know it then but I was obtaining wisdom beyond my years. I would gain momentum if I helped around the kitchen or at least around the area where the cooks hung out. I had longed to find meaningful friendships, and the fictional characters on tv made me feel hopeful that I would be able to make quality friends, just like regular people. I would pretend I was one of those characters I would see on the television. The telly tube had all of the answers that no one would answer. What to do when approached by a potential friend. What to say if you make a mistake. How to talk to boys. How to make cool friend groups.

Watching characters from Family Matters; Moesha, and Fresh Prince of Belar on tv gave me the courage to reach out and try to make friends. I Didn't have much luck finding quality friends . I chose quantity in school but wasn't shown much love. Some thought I was too awkward. Maybe they could see that I wasn't sure of myself. No one really wanted to hang around a nerd who loved Rock; Xmen, Rap, cloud watching, tree climbing, Reggae and mermaids. When life was great, I climbed trees, drank loads of porridge, layed on the grass and stared at the clouds. My imagination forever ran wild and

I didn't really have a care in the world, until I did. That my friends is called adulting. Adulting is hard. Have a plan; build on your goals or else life will write the script for you. I could tell my parents loved each other, the smiles and gentle touches. I remembered long after they wanted to forget.  Our home was filled with lots of love and food, until it wasn't. The home was filled with blame and resentment, It felt like I was a reminder of another thing they did wrong.  There once were smiles that turned to sorrow. An inevitable end. When I was young I wanted with all my heart to be normal. Even to my detriment. I didn't know that being normal is not the goal! Moving in the image in which you were made, is much more conducive to your health. Normality is a sham, a huge front. I didn't know what I know now. Doing everything in my power to appear as regular as humanly possible. I didn't do my own due diligence. Searching for who I was, instead of listening to others who haven't got a clue. As a human being who went through big trauma. I didn't speak up. I let myself be led astray and I was unfocused towards stability and actually living. Studies show 90% of Autistic women experienced sexual violence. I want this number to decrease dramatically. That's why I wanted to write this book. The more stories we hear about the better prepared we will be.

As a family we would enjoy meals together, participate in family gatherings, practice our faith, and had lots of fun together. I would read the bible with my grandmother, it slowed me down, grew my empathy and strengthened my relationship with GOD. I really appreciated my upbringing and was truly grateful for my parents, and all of our shenanigans together. I wished that there was more communication, more freedom to be ourselves instead of a well groomed version.  Life was good until it wasn't... False positivity can be very detrimental. Smile, don't feel, don't tell, keep quiet. Parental breakups can also affect children, and young people as well as the couple going through the break up. When my parents fell apart it hurt me real bad. I never voiced it, but it showed through strange actions.

**"We learn wisdom first, by reflection. Which is noblest. Second, by imitation which is easiest, and third by experience which is the bitterest." - Confucius**

Relationships were difficult for me to form. Being able to discern the wolves from the sheep was not easy for me. I was a very naive child and hated when others would point it out. I didn't realize my boundaries and limitations. I was impulsive and needy. The wrong people got to me which happens when your family is unraveling. I Didn't know that I was autistic and navigating communication and relationships was extremely difficult. I Had to maneuver around being called dumb blonde; white washed, stuck up. A black girl who is struggling to articulate herself is doomed; to forever be told she needs to get over herself; or my absolute favorite, "she's faking it." Could it be that there were other attributing factors that may be at play here?. No, NO, not that.!

Growing up, I had long natural hair, in grade school some students would pull my hair and ask if my hair was real. I didn't understand why people were so mean. I wanted to teach the world about differences, and uniqueness. We lived in Etobicoke, Martingrove and Eglington. I would write down my thoughts and grievances that I experienced or observed. You don't really see curious, peculiar black girls like me around those parts. I stuck out like a sore thumb. I'd practice what I might say, if confronted in a more confident assertive voice. I would turn on some music and dream about how many of the artists I would meet from Right

On Magazine, just because of my writing, just because I was doing great things in the world. I couldn't remember a lot of cool things to talk about usually so I would stay tuned in so I could conduct conversations with my research. I thought I knew the world I lived in. I would soon learn what the world is really about.

I loved radio, radio was like magic taking you to different places all at once. Finding out new and interesting information each time you turned the knob. When I used my pre-set lingo, persons could resonate with me because I used my encyclopedias, conducted research with my family and found ways to learn and adapt. Practicing in my room. It sounded like a monotone robot when I spoke but it worked. But for how long? I didn't know what it was, what was wrong or what was right with my brain but I had an idea that I was weird. Something was up, I wanted to be able to name it instead of others placing their labels unto me.

If I sat real, real still, and kept quiet. I could get away with being one of the gang, appearing to be like the others. You know the saying "the less you say, the smarter you look", well I found the phrase to be true but only for a short time. I used that to my advantage sometimes to get into the conversations around me, to feel a part of the group. Until someone wanted to call on me for being too quiet. Then my cover would be blown. I needed more time whatever it was either my teachers or my parents would assign for me to do.

My heart is filled with loads more feelings than the average person. I possess a high amount of feelings, I believe it's the feelings my parents withheld from each other got transferred to me. Some would say that I feel too much. Not a lot of people know about possessing immense emotions. Immense thoughts all at once, all the time. I am a beautifully complex creature. I recognized that I was different when I was about nine years old, I found it difficult to stay still or keep focus. "Oh Tasha it's okay you don't have to feel that way", " Natasha, you're reacting like you always do". Those comments drove me nuts. Stop testing me! Lighting me up, Tearing me down because of your own insecurities. When teachers started to do it I knew there was something there but I didn't have a name for it. I didn't understand. I'm me. But now, no more letting others that didn't do their own innerwork tear me down. No more intentional misunderstandings and my name at the heart of it. I'm not the cause of your problems, and if I was the issue  you can  come to me and discuss your grievances.

I realized how to work around others who refuse to grow. Others who refuse to take accountability for their behavior and negative treatment. Because advocating for myself wasn't second nature I would keep quiet when I needed to speak up. I was loud, even when I needed to keep quiet. Unregulated emotions look messy.

Life would not morph into something positive until I demonstrated I could be a contributing member of society. Living for God and doing what the Lord intended me to do in my life. Life shifted when I realized that traumatic events would follow me around if I didn't heal. Find peace and happiness in every inch of life. If you don't find the calm amongst your stormy heart, you will not find the peace that you seek.  I didn't have coping strategies to deal with burnout; sensory overload, or meltdowns. Once I had found the tools to deal with the array of issues that come with seen and unseen disabilities. I was able to breathe a little bit easier. Life shifted when I realized that I don't have to share my life with everyone.

It's okay to say no, or no thank you, and not provide a reason.

The word no can save your life. It's important to have boundaries when it comes to family and friends. They can run a muck if you let them. I don't have to adhere to everything that's said to me, I must use discernment. My intentions are genuine. I may be annoying to you, or weird but I love hard and play even harder. I give my all in relationships. Thank God I have much more understandings about how life is supposed to be lived. I have faith and ambition. In some situations that arose, I would ask for clarity and get shut down. Not many people will say they're sorry or attempt to right their wrong. Unless the person is a high value individual.

Unless the person values and respects me. Life shifted when I journeyed to become my true self even when it made others uncomfortable. Life turned when I chose to be obedient to God, learned from my past and created my own values, beliefs, boundaries, and learned to live by my values and boundaries. I delved deeper into identifying my disabilities, owning who I am and being okay with who I see in the mirror. Developing tools and structures that brought peace and joy into my life instead of disappointment and grief. I took time to investigate myself to decipher my differences and learned how to accept how my brain worked. My ADHD (Attention Deficit Hyperactivity Disorder) brain cleaned out every piece of junk that I would keep and carried around for over 20 years. I cleaned out all of the old clothes, and old papers that were stored up around my house . Every trinket and book that I no longer needed,I gave away or donated. I cleaned house, made room for the wonderful life God has in store for me. Made room to be filled with peace and love. Made room for forgiveness and consolidation. There is nothing that is going to stop me from achieving my goals which is to be great in God's eyes first before anyone else. I got things twisted and others around me never let me forget it. Now that I understand,

I will do better.  I've done the inner and outer work needed to not have to use more than one voice to get my point across, that's for all of my code swichers out there who know what i'm talking about. I can just be me ; ) without having to guess or wonder.  I will not shy away from what makes me unique. Life began to get better when I embraced my disabilities with love and treated myself with respect. Stay positive. Keep a sense of humor in difficult times. By doing this you'll spend less time worrying and more time executing.

In 2016, I was diagnosed with Autism and other diagnoses. I knew that I was different every ameba in my body told me so, now I could breathe much easier. I just didn't know why. But at that moment, everything that I had gone through made perfect sense. Everything started to all add up. My brain wasn't broken, my brain just works differently. I started to look into what autism meant.

What neurodivergence was, and how many others had excelled with autism. I finally had a reason for what and why I existed the way that I did, changed my life forever. I wished I had been diagnosed at an earlier age because it made such a difference. Not putting so much pressure on myself to be normal, be like everyone else. I wanted so badly to be like everyone else, I would put up with a tremendous amount of negativity from others around me just to fit in. Knowing why my nervous system was on overdrive all the time gave me the freedom to finally be ME. I need tremendous amounts of patience and kindness. Which I would seek from others. Now I show myself more patience and grace before anyone else.

# My suggestion to you:
# BE YOU PERIOD!! With no equivocation.

Constantly advocating to gain simple access to supports necessary to succeed. The plight of a person struggling to be heard, I guess. I want to be a changemaker in the realms of Education, Employment and Family. I struggled in these areas and I saw a lot of other parents and young people struggle as well. Personal bias and prejudice generally can influence the way one may think about a person. Personal bias, prejudice and ableism diminishes a person's abilities and disabilities. I was finally able to maneuver myself much more confidently in the world. I found my voice and creativity. They say that God doesn't make mistakes, and I knew then that this statement was a true fact, now it's time to start acting like I wasn't a mistake. Moving in the world with much more confidence and intention. I was made exactly how I was supposed to be made. Imperfectly perfect! As a mom with unseen disabilities, I wanted to share my journey of big and small traumas; to know who I am and becoming the woman I was meant to be with the world. I want to encourage and uplift another to make change in their lives.

I embraced my imperfections by creating a sweet and loving way to talk to myself. My disabilities are not my imperfections. Constantly trying to fit in and be normal was one of my imperfections. I had to learn to value what I had to say, period. One day I developed "CreateDon'tHate," which was born out of frustration—the frustration of people hating on people like me with seen or unseen disabilities.

I used CreateDon'tHate as an anthem to overcome tough times.

I decided to start a movement of my own that promotes hope, courage, and love through the CreateDon'tHate video podcast on YouTube.

"CreateDon'tHate" is a real practical way to build community and connection. I've had the chance to meet multiple high-value individuals along my journey, all because I choose to embrace my disabilities. There is a portrait in my home of a striped elephant, that I value so much because it signifies me as the striped elephant in the room. I stand in the room loud and proud and unapologetically me.

As someone who is Authentically Autistic, among other wonderful things, I embraced my imperfections by looking in the mirror and asking myself a couple of questions. How do I contribute to my own problems? What seeds do I plant for the future? Who do I have around me and why? Do they assist in my success or not? I embraced my imperfections by taking each breath with intention and being of service to others from my overflow, not from a depleted space. Stirring far from high control groups. And people who wish to keep me small for their own enjoyment. I believe acts of kindness can change anyone's perspective about their own lives. Embracing my imperfections looked like eating better, walking more, drinking more water, and speaking positively and with love towards myself every minute. I embraced my own imperfections by knowing and believing that I am wonderfully and powerfully made, and I know whose I am and who I am.

It's important to know whose you are because having a belief system changes the game significantly. Unseen Disabilities is a part of who I am. Unseen disabilities don't define me. I have value just as much as the next person, and so do you! Having faith can assist you in building a strong back bone to be able to handle what life throws at you. Giving your all to a higher being in order for the bigger battle to be won. Your peace of mind! Looking back, now I know if I had continued down the old path, listening to people who don't mean what they say and lie when you bring it up. People who constantly talk about your downfalls and won't ever let you get over not even one Fall. It's like they got used to throwing me under the bus. No area of my life was safe. I would have lived an unfulfilled life, if I didn't do my inner work! I Started to look at the plank in my own eye, unlike what the family and friends I had been around. What do we do? Not standing and advocating for yourself, opens the door for others to dictate your wants and needs, leaving you at the mercy of others. Some people don't know where they're going, or who they are, oftentimes those same people tend to draw others in like a magnet, and if you do not know yourself enough to withstand this force you will be pulled off your course, a path you were never intended to be on. Please don't listen to those people. Run away; flee, depart, separate, stay far from persons that do not respect or honor who you are and where you are intended to go.

***Earl Nightingale said, "Take a ship with no captain, no crew, no aiming point, no destination, or no guidance, no goal, and start the engines and let it go. I think you'll agree if it leaves the harbor at all, it will either sink or wind up on some deserted beach, at derelict".***

This quote tells me that we have to have intentional and specific goals, a deliberate destination or else you'll steer your ship into nothingness. In other words you'll steer your life into the gutter.

Looking back, I could've prioritized my mental wellness, sought out help for myself, and did not wait on others for assistance. I had gone through tough traumas, a large scab grew over my body in the form of debilitating shame. None of what happened to me was my fault but it sure felt like it was. I could've made more high-value relationships by first looking at myself as a valuable person. I needed to advocate for myself more to get what I needed and wanted in order to be a successful woman, someone advocating for me, and cheerleading for me showing me how to look at my disabilities as advantages not weaknesses. Having community would have helped even more. So, I say to you, just be you; that's all you can do.

Believe in your abilities; you must be willing to not care about what others think and prioritize joy, peace, love, grace, and happiness. Being okay with my unseen disabilities has taken me through the ringer. But I choose to participate in activities that bring proper meaning and true substance to my life and another's life as well. Surround yourself with authentic people who promote growth. Keep attune to how others make you feel and make adjustments accordingly. I was an accommodator. That's right I'll say it again, I was an accommodator! When I stopped accommodating I became more intentional for myself.

Again, saying no and prioritizing myself became a big part of my success. Pay attention to what activities drain you and which activities make you feel alive. Remember, we are all perfectly imperfect, and that's okay. There is nothing wrong with being different or awkward. As Issa Ray once said, "I'm Awkward and Black" That statement just sums me up in a nutshell. The journey to becoming me looked like accepting who I was, having deep faith, and understanding in Whose I was. When you know that you move differently, more confidently. Life is full and abundant.

*Fill your hearts with faith and the inner knowing of who you are. This will help you through the really rough journey called life. Plan your steps, so your gifts can shine through.*

# MY ABILITY IS MY STRENGTH
## By: MissNatasha

My ability comes from God

My ability is powerful

My ability is strong

My ability can create many things

My ability can change my world

I am able to dance

I am able to sing

I am able to do anything

I am able to pick up my toys

I am able to make noise

I am able to walk the dog

I am able to pick up a log

I am able to give a helping hand

I am able to make change in my community

I am able to create friendships that do not take away from who I am as a person

I am able to stay authentically me

I am able to LOVE Big

I am able to laugh

I am able to ask for what I need

I am able to talk to someone if I am feeling down

I am able to go for a walk or ride my bike

I am able to play hockey;

baseball, football or soccer if I like

I am able to sit in the sun and enjoy the breeze

I am able to read books and listen to the radio

I am able cry and express how I feel or what I think

I am able to voice my opinion

My ability is Great and Mighty

My ability will never run out of my abilities,

as long as I stick to my goals and vision

My abilities are not a Dis

My abilities are mine

My abilities are Me

# FEELINGS
## AREN'T FACTS
## SO FIND OUT THE
# FACTS
## SO YOU CAN SORT OUT
# YOUR FEELINGS
### -MissNatasha

# CHAPTER 2
# IN MY FEELINGS

Come as You Are; a 2019 movie about three young men with disabilities who hit the road to Montreal to lose their virginities. How brave, how exciting, how scary the journey must have been for these young men. These individuals wanted to travel to Montreal, where there is an establishment that caters to people with disabilities in a sexual way. This would give the young men an opportunity to lose their virginities. More than 80% of persons with Autism want to be in a romantic relationship with someone. A documentary following four Autistic people navigating love and romantic relationships shares the story of one young man who I deeply resonated with. This young man longed to have a companion but didn't know all it took to find; keep or maintain a relationship. To me, stories like this one are about self advocacy. These men and women possess bravery and the strength needed to venture out into the world, taking a chance to find what makes them happy. The greatest risk that we take is to be seen and heard for who we truly are! I know, I know, right but you're in for a treat with both of these films. And it's going to bring up a few talking points for you caregivers out there as well. What do we believe a grown man and woman with disabilities can and can't do? Does the individual have a say in their own lives? What is the protocol ???? Listening to others can be a double edged sword for persons with seen and unseen disabilities. You have to trust that the person's advice and guidance is coming from a genuine place and that the direction is in your best interest. If you're naive like myself, you could be talked into doing things that you don't feel comfortable doing.

An easy target, no one would be the wiser because the attitude is attributed to being a black woman not sexual trauma, not the masking, not the disabilities. Growing up a Canadian still didn't shield me from trauma. The negative gaze of people who think that they are better than you can be hidden, a covert way to keep someone small. Growing up and even into adulthood, I would notice how I'd be right on the money with certain things and way off the mark with others. I had no idea what Theory of mind was. How It differs from neurotypical and neurodivergent people, neurotypical to neurospicy. We are all made unique. I'd be mature in some senses. Like, knowing how to wash and fold clothes at a certain age. But not being able to cook certain other foods because of the smell or feel of the items involved in creating the dish. Theory of mind is the ability to recognize the intentions of others. The fact is not all neurodivergent persons have difficulty with others intentions or beliefs. Sometimes we are manipulated into thinking that our thoughts or beliefs are wrong for another person's gain. Sometimes we miss expressions or emotions. There are some like me who have heightened senses; immense emotion. I choose not to go into detail of things that happened to me because we all have sad songs, violin songs. Sorrowful times in life that we can't take back. Experiences that shaped us into the people that we are today. Good or bad. Did you let your violin songs ruin your life or fuel your life into greatness? We have a choice to nurture those around us or tear them down. I was in my feelings about so many of my family and friends who had a gaze. Only when it came to me or my offspring. When I started to take my own thoughts and feelings seriously before others. Things got real. When you're involved in relationships like these it's best to speak up about your wants and needs immediately. Don't wait, don't be silent! Speaking up right as the violations occur can weed out the positive and negative people in your life. We may have difficulty determining between an individual's actions but patterns don't lie.

*Almost all people gain at least some of their sense of self - worth by how people perceive them.  -David Smeenk 2023*

Just the gaze of an angry black woman looking for attention, looking for a handout. Self Advocacy is defined as the action of representing oneself or one's views and interests. Asking for assistance; asking for what you need and using assertive communication. As someone who is authentically autistic advocating for myself wasn't always second nature. Most of my life I heard or was made to feel, I was insufficient or Not Enough. Stay obedient! Listen and take heed! But take heed to who? And when am I allowed to have my own values, beliefs and traditions? How do you build strong foundations? When do you heed to your own values and ambitions? Caribbean parents are also Sons and Daughters; Uncles and Aunties, Friends and Lovers. In some homes we don't get to hear the stories of old that could have helped us. Whether it be menopause; or sex, how to say no or how to take no for an answer. We need to do better as a whole and stop playing perfect. There is only one and HE is not made like us!

Growing up I had others tell me what to think because for some reason my words were not valid. I'd obey even when I knew better. I needed an interpreter. But you know what I realized after some time that we all have an interpreter embedded into our bodies and you want to know what that is called? The Holy Spirit. I had a compass inside of me the whole time. Didn't know how to access it but at the most RUFFest times it activated something inside of me that reminded me of where I came from. Reminding me WHOSE I was. I'd still believe the other person had more authority. When there is only One authority.

When I spoke up, about what I was being told or my own thoughts on matters I was met with upset, I didn't listen to my first mind. I conformed! I surrendered to the whims of others. Their power and ego trips.

## Access Self Advocacy through Self Knowledge

My first mind, my intuition would tell me something. There are internal pressures that occur under the surface. I will be rejected. I will not find loving friendships, our family dynamics. My circle was supposed to be safe and most would tell me I shouldn't think like that, or you are thinking too hard. But they were the ones violating of course they would invalidate my feelings, some kind of sick game.

# Points to remember:

# (Lynne Soraya, 2013, Author of Living Independently on the Autism Spectrum)

- Start by being your own friend, learn to be a friend to yourself first

- Assess why you want to have a relationship with someone, I will go on to even say any relationship. Don't feel pressured to pursue a relationship just because "everyone else does"

- Relationships require all of the skills that friendships do. Be sure to think about the future

- Like yourself first, people notice. Decide ahead of time what traits you want to seek in a friend

- Don't get too close to a friend too quickly

- Remember that transitions in life happen, your social circles will change, you may grieve, but don't take it personally. Some people aren't for you

- Avoid exploitative people, friends should be concerned with your feelings and respect them

Sometimes you know that the person; place or thing isn't for you. We'll still mess around and eat a pack of sugar cookies, instead of just eating one or three. We gotta recognize that just because of another's opinion, we don't have to change our opinion to accommodate or please others. Especially the one who are intentionally involved in misunderstanding you and putting you and your abilities down. There are people in and around your life that don't deserve the amount of effort you put in. None of your energy! You have to learn how to discern who the right people are in your own life. Be mindful of this and store the energy for the really rough and tough times. Store your energy for people who respect and love you without hate or put downs. The individuals who deserve each and every second of your energy will be there after the smoke clears, they don't have a self righteous disposition. Our differences are not all of who we are and if someone fails to see it don't push the agenda.

I started to rebel and disconnect from my core values, straying into the darkness. Hanging around people; places and things that were Not for me. Having a sense of belonging is an important thing. I wish I knew and loved the positive traits about myself. I wish it wasn't sniffed out and stomped on. I was that cheerleader always wanting the best for you. Our image is classified as socially acceptable if you can mainstream your appearance. There are basic rules and regulations that female friendship groups adhere to. I am here to say that I am bound to the light and freedom in living correctly. No more conformity. In grace filled peace! I was so overwhelmed by the repetitive comments and unsolicited advice, and comments. So I conformed. Doing like everyone else is most deadly. As an autistic individual we are made to accommodate regular people in every aspect of our lives. It's like you gave up. It's like you don't care. It's like you waving your white flag. If you didn't know conformity is a recipe for disaster.

## Sometimes we mistake our most immeasurable gifts for shameful flaws

I found joy and peace in building my faith and understanding in Whose I was, and how much I had to do in this world. My faith and acts of service kept me grounded and in constant reflection. Be okay in the skin that was given to you. Take pride in every quirk.

What happens when you don't self advocate? By not advocating for yourself; you can get taken advantage of. I myself had been taken advantage of on several occasions and nothing was done about it. I felt discombobulated; at times weakend emotionally, and extremely depressed. I went quiet in 2016, asking God to give me the courage and wisdom to find the voice I once muted. What I found in return out weighted anything that may come up. Things changed even more for me in 2017, I started to realize my worth. Figure out where I belonged. It was difficult and scary but worth it. I understood that if I stayed quiet and let others advocate for me. I would be living normally, like everyone else! That just wasn't something I was comfortable doing anymore. I had been born to stand out and spread sunshine across the land. I started to live authentically me, autistically me. To me this is absolutely the way to authenticity and self advocacy. At one time or another I realized that I hummed to calm myself, get back to the center.

If overstimulated; overwhelmed or frustrated, I'd humm. Some persons on the spectrum make all sorts of noises. Some are completely silent, by choice or not. We are all different and wonderfully made. It is more isolating when you try to fit in, instead of standing out like you were born to do. If you find yourself feeling scared or apprehensive about advocating for yourself try going out in nature to ground yourself again. Make an intentional decision for yourself on your own problem. Find that real voice inside, what is it you've wanted to do?

Find a supportive group, encourage and uplift you. A place where you can feel safe to communicate your thoughts honestly and openly. Your life will be much more worthwhile over time if you believe in your gifts and strengths.

I cared what others thought; I was groomed to, I was manipulated to, I chose too. Some Autistic individuals make easy targets for manipulation. In a 2015 survey, 80% of Autistic individuals indicated that they had been taken advantage of by someone they thought was a friend. Have you heard of the phrase MateCrime? It's a term that is prevalent to persons with disabilities, especially Autism. Perpetrator befriends a vulnerable person with the intention of exploitation. Experiencing pain or discomfort when in friendships or relationships and family dynamics so many times I started to do research on what I was experiencing. Finding myself in situations with others, that books say are not good for your health. I had to write about the experiences, in order to help someone else. Someone else could resonate and change their own trajectory by leaning on God. Do you know what is an essential part of a balanced diet? Being your authentic self! Create Don't Hate!

If you don't advocate for yourself, you'll live an unfulfilled life, people will dictate your wants and needs for you and you'll be at the mercy of others. Underemployed; difficulties in school, difficult to make high value relationships, prioritize your mental wellness by advocating for yourself! We were made to each individually do something great in the world, in doing so you will uplift another. Being your authentic self is a great part of a well balanced breakfast; lunch and dinner! To be your most authentic self you've gotta be willing to **NOT** care what others think. I had an absolute problem with that. Because I was caught up in TOP TEAR PEOPLE

PLEASING. **<u>I absolutely 1000% percent don't recommend this!</u>**

Believe in yourself and your abilities. Don't allow the negative gaze of another to stir you from your true self. Guilt; shame, and low self esteem start when you're untrue to yourself. When you negate the slight tap on the shoulder that the holy spirit is giving you.

That silent push in the other direction. That, Hello, are you there???? I am trying to get your attention on this matter and you don't want to listen. Listen!

Start with asking yourself; what do I value? How do I want to show up in the world? Keep attune to who you are with and how others make you feel. What types of activities do you have to do in a day ? Which activities make you feel alive and which activities drain you. Prioritize joy; peace, love, grace, happiness, activities that bring meaning and true substance. Surrounding yourself with authentic people can promote growth and authenticity.

Thank you very much for reading this book, it's much appreciated. I didn't value my voice, my opinion wasn't valued. I wanted others who have gone through similar thought processes to have an understanding of another. Someone like me, others have labeled you before even knowing who you really were. Someone who has a lot of what I call violin songs coming out the wazoo. Violin songs are Tramas. When you have tramas it gives the people around you silent permission to deal with you dirty. Give help but invoice you invisible receipts. Rotten like. Then blame you for being who you are without rhyme nor reason. They just seem to get away with dogging you out and not apologizing for it. Getting away from that requires planning; valuing yourself, and boundaries.

# Teach people how to treat you!

For some reason they feel as though this behavior is okay because you play nice, you play small in their game. It's been a long, ass road. I'm not all at fault and I refuse to continue carrying the negative gazes of others.

We should be able to love and authentically care for one another instead of avoiding or judging. We deserve to rest and live in peace. I will forever generously forgive because that's what I would want my Lord to do for me. Someone once said. When a person you loved deeply, did you the dirtiest. It changes you. You need a higher power to bring you back to reality. My intention is to enlighten you to express your own individual self advocacy, self love, towards yourself first because you're no use if your own grass is all dry up and crusty. I wanted to share something from the bookBradshaw on: The Family, Dr John Bradshaw, studied shame and family dynamics. Dr. Bradshaw says, shame is a kind of a soul murder. Shame is a sickness of the soul.

I started my academic journey in 2003. A seemingly scary and new experience. I have had situations arise where I've spoken to the professors and was told I should just keep quiet, there was no need to make any noise or ruckus. And disrespect is a part of working in groups and we have to learn how to deal with it. Those comments kept me at bay for a while. Disheartened and alone, enduring situations like constantly being ignored, eye rolling asking me to be in a group then totally leaving my name out of the agenda of the group workshop assignment was something I had to DEAL with alone. Alone is what I felt! So I started to do my research. I found that many organizations have words on their walls and policies in binders but it's all fake, a farce. I would remember walking by hallways where this particular institution had plaques hanging on the wall stating how they are inclusive of everyone!

Create Don't Hate! We must continue to speak about the injustices occurring within our workspaces; in our homes and within our schools.

That is why I started NatashaConnects which is based on M.E.E.F, Mental Wellness within Education Employment and Family. Providing tools and strategies to cultivate Mental Wellness within Education, Employment and Family through books, workshops, speaking engagements etc. I was melting away and needed to Creatively heal whilst extending the resilience of another in a creative and thoughtful way. Hence this book. I believe books to be one of those avenues to clarity. To greater understanding. It is difficult to maintain friendships. I was glorified "blurred" Black nerd. Repeated rejection or negative reactions from others can take a toll. It could have been because I talked about the library or what book I have gotten.

No one understood my plight. The people who I thought I could trust betrayed my trust and confidence. Leaving me feeling more alone and isolated than ever. I was all advocated out, tired and drained. Drained from others' ignorance, I never asked you to feel sorry for me. Disgusted by the behaviors of others. It's sad to see that the people that I trusted the most choose to treat me in underhanded ways. Handing out invisible receipts for so-called good deeds. I grew saddened and defeated. My grades suffered because of the unsafe environments and experiences I've had throughout my time in school. But I didn't let that stop me. I thought professors;

school administrators, counselors, supervisors, managers, aunts, uncles, cousins, coworkers are there to help, not hinder.

I did not want to admit that I socially struggled to the degree that I had. I had no thought in my mind to share with anyone growing up. I vigorously wanted to conceal my flaws; and struggles to understand. I would imitate my surroundings to go undetected, this tactic only lasted a short period of time. I didn't get very far socially. Tony Attwood, in his book The Complete Guide to Asperger's Syndrome spoke about " God Mode " Where the person ends up creating a persona in order to face the world. I would go into God Mode, No room for mistakes! I was confused with the intentions of what someone would be dealing with. I grew an attitude and started to malfunction. Pretending to understand what was going on in group conversations. I would pretend I had friends growing up and write letters that my pretend friends would send me. Asking me questions about who I was and what I liked to do , instead of only doing what the other person wanted to do. I'd observe the mannerisms of another person greeting or meeting someone. Then cross reference the interaction. The disingenuous nature of the interactions I was having with people close to me, didn't make sense. I realized people have choices and biases. My attempts to fit in somewhere always ended with someone in the social group finding out that there is something about that girl. They'd start to ramp up pointing and making fun more often. Sooner or later they ghost and that's that. I desperately wanted to be someone else. But the best person you can be is yourself. We should not be thirsting after superficial social acceptance. This behavior kills! Murders your soul! When it's all over they will say bad things about you. It's never worth it, compromising your self worth for others. All I had to do was accept myself wholeheartedly. No social status. No social acceptance. I have had a considerable amount of time allocated to pleasing people, which led to the melting of my brain. Sometimes we only realize our brains are melting when its too late and years have passed. I needed a reset. Some sort of emergency switch. I started to gather up the materials to construct a white flag. That took a couple more years. I started to notice the power trips others close to me would play with me. I sickened my stomach! Even up until today. I started to speak up and set parameters around what I will and will not tolerate. If I voiced a real opinion about something or another that didn't put other people first or I was thinking too big for my tiny self. THey would build clicks with others around me to make themselves feel superior. They didn't come to me and talk about it. I am not sure why, maybe its because they were afraid to hurt me or a combination of pride and ego. But silence is still communication! This is why I share my stories and question everything someone tells me. With my knowledge and lived experiences I can assist another in stirring away from these types of people in their own lives. An overwhelming whirlwind.

# Self Affirmations, by: Liane Holliday Willey (Willey 2001, pg. 164)

- I am not defective, I am different

- I will not sacrifice my self worth for peer acceptance

- I am a good and interesting person

- I will take pride in myself

- I am capable of getting along with society

- I will ask for help when I need it

- I am a person who is worthy of others' respect and acceptance

- I will find a career interest that is well suited to my abilities and interests

- I will be patient with those who need time to understand me

- I am never going to give up on myself

- I will accept myself for who I am

These 5 Affirmations mean more to me than the others, they are all important don't get me wrong. When I realized the importance of being yourself and loving every curve, every flaw unconditionally I believe it was too late. I hope that you can be the very best you can be regardless of who says. I don't have to sacrifice who I am to be accepted. I had learned this at a later age but I will not regret the journey.

Despite what my family says, I am an interesting and loveable person and I don't have to do what they say or act as they act in order to be accepted.

- **I will not sacrifice myself worth for peer acceptance**
- **I am a good and interesting person**
- **I am a person who is worthy of others' respect and acceptance**
- **I will be patient with those who need time to understand me**
- **I am never going to give up on myself**

# BECAUSE I'M A BLACK WOMEN
## BY: MISSNATASHA

Because I'm a black woman you don't think you have to apologize

Because I'm a black woman you think it's okay not to greet me

Because I'm a black woman I know how to apologize

Because I'm a black woman there's a tinge, a sound to your voice that you only do with me

Because I'm a black woman you think you can miss handle, and miss use me

Because I'm a black woman you think I could you could stereotype me I miss treat me

Because I'm a black woman, he think that you could string me along

Because I'm a black woman, it's okay for you to not resolve your issues with me

Because I'm a black woman

Because I'm a black woman, you think I have no value in your eyes

Because I'm a black women, you think I have too much strength

Because I'm a black woman, you think I shouldn't have power

Because I'm a black woman you think I can't be blessed just as you are

Because I'm a black woman you believe what people say

Because I'm a black woman, you perpetuate what society says

Because I am a black woman you don't think you have to try

Because I'm a black woman, your ignorance remains bliss

Because I'm a black woman you don't admit when you're wrong

Because I'm a black women you find it funny to scapegoat

Because I'm a black women you think is okay to blame and shame

Because I'm a black women you use my ideas and don't give me credit

Because I'm a black women you feel uncomfortable to talk to me, get to know me

Because I'm a black women you want me around for photo opts

Because I'm a black women your scared

Because I'm a black women you say I'm a bad mother

Because I'm a black women you pronounce my name wrong

Because I'm a black women you don't pick up the phone

Because I'm a black women you ignore me

Because I'm a black women it's easy to makeup a story

Because I'm a black women you never tell the true story, the real story

Because I'm a black women you use me for my time

Because I'm a black women you don't see me relaxed

Because I'm a black women your gaze is different towards me compared to another

Because I'm a black women you believe there is no reason to smile

Because I'm a black women I'll continue to smile

Because I'm a black women

THE COMFORT ZONE IS THE ENEMY OF COURAGE AND CONFIDENCE

-Brian Tracey

# CHAPTER 3

# LEARNING CONSISTENCY AND CLIMBING MOUNTAINS

Erykah Badu's song "Bag Lady" was a hit in 2000, the lyrics rocked the souls of many who were not doing the inner work. Erykah sings, "One day all 'em bag goin' get in your way" Some would say that I was a bag lady with all of the drama that I would carry around. Not only was I carrying baggage, I was holding onto other people's baggage as well. Wearing labels that others had assigned to me. Very detrimental practice, not recommended for anyone. I started really carrying hockey bags of baggage when I thought that I could make friends in Ridge. They tricked me. They set me up. I was lost for a good while after that. I learned that I allowed others to bamboozle me. I made them trick me. I gave permission and accommodated the disrespect.

## Shed them bags sweet heart!
## Leave them bags alone.

How do I know that I am to blame you ask, well I'll let you in on what I learned. How difficult and tough it would be to climb a mountain with heavy baggage. Reputation is what others think you are. Character is what you really are! How difficult would it be to go to a ball with a whole hockey bag full of stuff! That doesn't look cute. Baggage can affect your whole life. You have to love and respect yourself before you can love and care for another person. Be a friend to yourself first! Do yourself a favor and let go.

I learned that telling your family every problem that occurs in your personal life before you've thought on your own problem first and prayed about it is not a good thing. That;s what Jesus and pets are for. I haven't really had pets before but I sure know that they aren't like people!!! I learned as a mother to be more attentive to my values and what you hold dear. As an Autistic black mother, I had individuals talk about my parenting; housekeeping, relationship etc. CONSTANTLY! I was such a downer. A let down that person's I hold dear would be like that.

I learned that some do not like to be seen for who they are but like to point out all of another's shortcomings. But it's scary to see how many would jump at the opportunity to point out or talk about my shortcomings. We must remember that all of us fall short in one way or another and there are determining factors for each and every one of our lives.

## Collaboration over Competition!

I learned that if you have a sense of faith in something and determination to bring about change in your life you can accomplish anything. I learned that if you keep your faith strong and be a faithful stewards, you will find life much easier to grow and flourish inside and out. I actually have accomplished a tremendous amount of my dreams. I am absolutely not going to stop living out the rest of my incredible dreams! I found that within the areas of Education, Employment and Family there was push and pull. I felt like I had little to say in the matter of my own life. Shedding the emotional baggage we carry will make the journey much, much easier, traveling up the mountain of life. Through the trenches of experience. Being a mother and a play wife not conducive for a young black woman with unseen disabilities. Don't ever play dolly house with anyone! Don't ever think that you won't encounter trials and tribulations.

## To climb mountains we have to be prepared.

But who prepares us for marriage and motherhood? Who do you go to for advice on boundaries and scapegoats? Who do you ask when you missed a step and you need sound advice? Some people come from families that had great, positive examples of marriage and parenting. Since the beginning of my time, I've taken risks; tried new things and stepped out of my comfort zone. Yet it's usually neurotypical people that have a hard time opening up their minds to new ways of thinking and interacting. I tried dating once or twice but I truly either showed too much of myself. I was rejected for, showed too little of myself or run or completely immersed in the other person's life, losing my sense of self. Which is never good. Others take examples from television shows or daydreams. Not necessarily! Start with your circle and build out from there. If not, find upstanding lawful people that you look up to to find your inspiration. Knowing exactly how to keep a relationship a float or set boundaries with others is important for long term friendships and partnerships to flourish. We bumped into one another at a very young age, fell in lust and had no blueprint for what the future would look like. Try and remember who you say "Hi" to! It may cost you more than you're willing to give. Take time to get to know one another and each other's strengths and weaknesses.

We had no foundation and didn't really talk about the plans for the future. Relationships are more difficult when you don't do your inner work. When you have unhealed people around you. When you haven't had professional help when you should have. Getting into a relationship as an autistic individual, make sure you have a great circle around you that is welcoming and grace filled. A circle who isn't going to talk about your life in a funny HaHa sort of way. Condescending in nature and going nowhere. Just like when I at home I became someone else's helper. Whatever that means? The housekeeper of the home worked contract jobs. I was not the main provider.

My flaw is not landing a full time job. Not being looked at as a viable candidate started to show up in every aspect of my life. I never landed a full time position. Who would take me? Statistics show that individuals with seen and unseen disabilities have a hard time finding and keeping employment. So in 2018 I decided to start my own business. I started from scratch, NatashaConnects, is a Mental Wellness and Disability Advocacy community. Building creative healing into the fabric of everything we do. It all starts with Create Don't Hate, a show and way of life around these parts! I live and breathe Creating Instead of Hating. Why you might ask? Because that is one thing no one can take from me! Creating instead of hating can't be taken from anyone because it's a way of life. A mindset. In relationships; friendships, Collaborations, Workplaces and families. Create Instead of Hate!

There are some who find relationships and love and there are some who don't. I landed into both categories. I wanted relationship with people so bad as a youth I ended up in trouble. And when I didn't really want relationship, just friendship I found something bigger, much scarier. I wanted to avoid marriage! Nope not for me, Thank YOu! Don't get me wrong when with the right person marriage is beautiful. I just didn't care for the stereotypical behaviours seen in real life and in movies. The "You know I LOVVVEEE's Yaaaaaaaaa" ; "Baby, Baby, Baby" The trash talk they give to their family and friends then wanna love on you in private. Rewiring the thought processes of old took me a long time to get through and I'm grateful. Now it's time to start real life with real people!

Society has taught us to believe that a woman can turn her house into a home. At some points in my life when I was struggling there were some signs that showed, and it showed around my home, I would be made fun of and talked about behind my back. They would literally come by to search and see. This was so infuriating because I couldn't quite understand the intentions of another but it usually showed up in another form. Ask God for wisdom. The wisdom to see the persons around you for who they truly are. This will help in the process towards climbing tall mountains or dealing with individuals who are fake and lack realness. Mountains will always be there. But the types of tools you gain or learn about along the way is very important. These tools will equip you. Create multiple avenues of creative healing: Eg: Arrange flowers in your home. Plant outdoors or indoors; wear a soft and fuzzy something, make a vision board. Color, doodle or dance. The goal is to lower anxiety levels down making it easier to engage with the world. Move that body. Movement moves emotions. Dance, put on some music, loosen up, even if just in your living room. Transmute your suppressed emotion into repetitive action, chopping wood, boxing, knitting, sewing. Expressive writing. Tools help you make sense of the world. Be more organized when stressors come up.

# I'M TIRED OF MEN

## BY: MISSNATASHA

Tired of men laughing at one another

Tired of men fighting one another

Tired of Fake men

Tired of pretentious men

Tired of manipulative men

Tired of men who don't care and lie like they do

Tired of men who don't tell you the real truth

Tired of gatekeeping men

Tired of men who think they're too much

Tired of men who are unsupportive

Tired of men who don't have faith

Tired of men who say they are one thing and do another

Tired of the men

Tired of men not owning up to their mistakes

Tired of men who say they care but have a funny way of showing it

Tired of men who don't support one another

Tired of men who think there too good to apologize

Tired of men who don't have respect

Tired of men who can't be respectful

Tired of men who talk too much and don't know what they are talking about

Tired of men who didn't do their own work!

Tired of men without consideration

Tired of men who steal

Tired of men who steal others time; soul, spirit

Tired of men who don't love themselves!

Tired of men who don't know how to behave

Tired of men can't be trusted

Tired of men who can't be trusted with important jobs

Soo, tired of men who don't appreciate an autistic women like me but take my ideas; my style, my cadence, my love, words, my care, my thoughts, misconstrue them and abuse them.

## WE CAN'T BECOME WHAT WE WANT BY REMAINING WHAT WE ARE

### -Max DePree

# CHAPTER 4

# LISTEN TO THE GOLDEN COMPASS BETWEEN YOUR EARS, YOUR BRAIN!

What is a compass? Well, a compass is a device that indicates direction. The compass is the most important instrument for navigation. The Golden compass is a children's book. The main character is given a compass with abilities beyond measure. The compass was called The Alethiometer. The Alethiometer, represents children's ability to discern truth. Just like life the truth isn't always black or white. For some autistic people we absolutely would have benefited from having someone to assist us from an early age. Someone who could help navigate the world and what's in store. The Golden compass assists the viewer in discerning the truth. There's so much going on in there at lightning speed. Deciphering it with a decoder, someone who can interpret the world for you as you go. Would be helpful but we don't live in that kind of a world as yet.

The Strangest Secret in the World, a book that I have read talks about the Golden Compass between your ears. Which part of your body do you think the book was referring to? Well if you guessed the brain you are right. The book The Strangest Secret in the World is referring to the active use of your brain, in a positive manner each and everyday. The use of your brain in strategic ways for your aspirations and worthwhile goals. If you are not using your brain in constructive and creative ways you are wasting your life away. When you creatively heal and use your brain space for solving important issues. You guarantee a greater success rate in your life.

*"WHEN YOU CREATIVELY HEAL YOU FREE UP MORE BRAIN POWER AND GIVE YOURSELF A FIGHTING CHANCE IN LIFE." -MissNatasha*

The healing is in how creative you are with your body; mind and soul. Listening to Earn your Leisure the other day and the hosts of the show always say heal your financial tramas before engaging with the financial world again. Creatively heal. Take time to notice what you think about; talk about most of the time. Be aware and conscious, the things we say out loud does have an effect. The music we listen to or the social media we intake. Live colorfully you. Vibrantly you! Having only good things to say to yourself is important. How do you function when you're unwell? How do you function when you're well? What are the creative steps that you take to get back to "normal"? Do you know what your normal looks like? Dismantle this narrative! You have value and worth, that doesn't look like anyone else's. Live in that beauty, fill yourself with all the reasons why your peace, patience and purpose is worth it. When the world deliberately mistreats you, misdiagnoses you, mismanages and misunderstands you. The best thing to do is go inward.

Find those creative ways to build yourself back up. Healing from the inside out. Do the backwards work. Take time to write, take pictures, vlog your experiences in order to learn more about your authentic self in order to gain a more broader creative perspectives of healing. I'll give you all an example of how I creatively healed.

I had been pretending to be regular for a long, long time. Keeping in the back of my mind that it is better to conceal instead of feel. But what you sweep in the closet or under the rug will come out as the largest ravenous dust bunny you've ever seen. Very, very hard to dust or clean up.  Well I have several stories from how I gained full access to my own thoughts and opinions. I avoided being my most authentic self because others around me. I didn't know that it was okay to fall or make mistakes. Well anyway, I started to go into nature, finding peace and inner quiet. I would ask the lord to reveal to me why I gravitate to certain people. Why I resonate with the very thing that I despise. Why do I react negatively to their negative reactions? How I can take back my power. I learned about God's love and appreciation.

I learned about the inner tools necessary to be free from negative people; places and things that had a deep hold over me. I started to love myself and how I was made purposefully. I started to speak up and speak out whenever there were disrespectful comments and behaviors. This process was extremely taxing, and only with a full understanding of Whose I was did I overcome and surpass the painful truths that being assertive and intentional with your life brings. I feel aware and whole. I am the grown and ready for what life has to offer, type of woman.

Creative healing can decrease anxiety; depression, negative self-worth, and a negative social identity. We are able to rearrange the frequencies in our brain to build better neural pathways for better brain function. Creativity isn't optional, creativity is necessity for my health. Art assists us to express the hard things, use it at home to bring about peace and creativity. Visual Arts is a great avenue for self expression. Focusing more on positive life experiences. Increased self-worth and identity by creating opportunities to overcome challenges, grow, and reach personal achievement. Positive social identity by not letting their illness define them. Expression of feelings in a symbolic way when words are difficult.

# THEY LAUGH AT US

## BY: MISSNATASHA

They laugh at us with their coworkers and colleagues

They make fun of how much we know compared to how much we don't know

They think that it's okay to not be heard or seen

They think it's okay to push off our priorities and our purpose

They think that we can't see or hear

They hear our cries and ignore each tear

They laugh at us and think that our hurts are Insignificant

They tell us to be quiet and don't say a word, when we need to do the opposite

They stifle our creative self esteem

They laugh at us when they use us for mindless labor but don't use our strengths

They laugh at us when we can't communicate our wants or needs

But are we letting them?

# Dr. John Bradshaw,( 1990)
# - Bradshaw on the Family (pg. 3)

**Emergence of False self:** Experiencing self is painful, thus a false self is born, conscientiously created. A defensive Mask which distracts from the hurt and pain. Years of pretending one can lose connection with who one really is. Your true self is numbed out.

# CHAPTER 5

# ALL MASKS ASIDE; TIME TO TALK ABOUT MASKING

Masking, the art of covertly disguising one's autistic traits to conform to societal norms, masking is a survival mechanism, a shield. Allowing a minimal amount of people to see our real unmasked self. Protecting us from being seen as different, or peculiar. Unlike the dominant default, the regular degular. Masking is often adopted by persons on the spectrum. But you can also find individuals masking out there in the world. At work; a woman of colour has to mask in unsafe work environments all the time. Newcomers from another country have to quickly mask in order to survive. If you're a black or brown Autistic individual you'll be taunted with the torment of having to prove yourself constantly, within all areas of your life. Having to perform a delicate dance balancing the expectations of negative cultural norms, that you don't even fit into. Continuing to wear layers and layers of masks over the years becomes even more complex. When viewed through the lens of intersectionality, we layer even more masks on. Being a black and brown woman; living with unseen disabilities, being different is not always celebrated.

Examples of masking in my life?

Observing the societal view of what is suggested black women should be and mimicking the look and nuance of that black women look different as the years moved on. Before 10 years old I was doing my very best to be the perfect girl. In EVERYONE's eyes. 10-13 yrs I went into a hip hop/ reggae confident phase. I wanted to have the lyrics at the ready, like an artist. I wanted to be able to take care of my family with my words. I wanted to make a difference in the world. Masking helped me but in the short term. Like sugar or a salty treat. It only satisfies your soul in a small period of time. No long term satisfaction comes from masking, masking is like something you're supposed to use when you go to court or something. "THey" always had an opinion! I had no idea how to turn off the sound. Too black or brown for some. Too white for others.  I found a mesh between Bashment girl and Hip-Hop head as a tween and teen. Preppy and sophisticated in some aspects of my life but no nonsense attitude. I felt too restricted in being my authentic self. I would act out with regards to my clothing and how I dressed. Influenced by color and fashion. I'd be ridiculed for my choices or befriended so "they" could take what I had and pretend that I was out of my mind.  I would display a facsimile of mish- mash up of parts appointed to me by others. Most times unable to convey freely some of the things I wanted to say. I grew up in many places around Toronto. Most times as a black or brown person it was frowned upon to be well spoken, intelligent, to love books and talk about certain topics. I presented in a lowly and modified manner. Sinking my soul, the very parts of me that were meant to shine. I noticed that when I spoke up about the way someone handled me, I was met with protest. I stopped trying to take off my masks. Reconnecting with my true self, being unapologetically and Autististically Me, Autistically Yours. The Lord doesn't want us to waste our gifts. We were made to give others encouragement in our own special ways.

Without self awareness and self acceptance, you can become lost. I'm aware of my limitations. I don't appreciate how many people assume otherwise! When communicated limitations within a safe environment one can feel at ease because the receiver of this information will be aware of how you operate.

# Emotional blackmail is a dysfunctional form of manipulation.

Some will try to emotionally manipulate you into staying compliant, stay small, keep on your mask. This is why it is imperative to deprogram your mind. No human is your master. Act accordingly! The thing is, any undercover would tell you. You can lose yourself if you aren't grounded in Whose you are and Who you are. Black and brown people have been led to believe that even within our own homes we must code-switch. Example of this is going to a family function wearing clothes that is deemed inappropriate. You go to Thanksgiving or Christmas dinner with your hair natural and there is a tremendous amount or comment on if everything is okay with you. Let us be. We have enough to deal with.

*Masking is how neurodivergent people navigate a neurotypical world. They may mimic social behaviors that are deemed more "socially acceptable" in neurotypical culture. (The Color of Emotional Intelligence by: Farah Harris, 2023)*

The need to mask ourselves becomes a coping mechanism, driven by the desire to avoid potential stigmatization and discrimination. I appointed myself head ambassador of mistakes and violations you're not supposed to make as an autistic individual.

Adaptive morphing, another word for masking or Camouflaging behaviors, **I do not mask to deceive!** I mask to survive and thrive. We live in a socially threatening world. For some with Autism, we fear the same old same old.

# Farah Harris displayed these examples of masking?

- Forcing eye contact

- Imitating facial expression and gestures

- Coping body language or tone

- Internalizing sensory discomfort

- Suppressing stimming (rocking, tapping etc)

- Pretending to understand or follow a conversation

- Rehearsing or scripting conversations

- Suppressing the desire to discuss intense interests or hyperfixations

I learned to find the appropriate things to discuss, didn;t always land but did a good enough job. Muting and re-muting myself to keep the peace. Giving excuses for my outbursts within every conversation. Erasing the very fabric of what made me, me! I'd share a fascinating fact at the wrong times. I got really excited when I saw the moon and I was waiting in line somewhere at night. Which was really annoying to some. While masking can provide a temporary shield against judgment, it comes at a cost. The internal struggle for authenticity becomes a constant companion. In her chapter Aspie Do's and Don't dating, relationships and Marriage. Hit the milestones that are widely accepted by friends and family.

Masking would help me to attract the perfect potential partner to keep family and friends at bae. Boyfriend; marriage, children, and so on. Would keep them quiet.  But unfortunately I believed false myths like these for decades. From: (pg.97) of Aspergers and Girls, Jennifer McIlwee Meyers (2016), chapter- Aspie-Do's and Don,'t: Dating, Relationships and Marriage.

Asperger's and Girls coauthor - Jennifer McIlwee Myers (2016) gave a great example of myths that we as persons with Aspergers may believe because of what we've seen on tv or we were told.

- The way to get yourself a man is to be feminine or dress in a certain way.

- Act like the kind of person that guys want and you'll get a guy

- Men are afraid of smart women who speak their minds

Dressing for the other person is not a good idea at all. No way negating how you want to enter the world isn't the ideal way to enter a relationship either. Be yourself! I've had some questionable attire over the years, trying to prove myself to people that didn't even matter.  I had a very hard time figuring out who I was and how to maneuver myself in this world. I was very friendly and curious. I wanted to know everything and wanted to be included in everything.

Had a long stint of staring, staring at others for long periods of time. I had an obsession with what made others tick. How did God make these differing human beings? I'd be caught as a child staring at my mother and father, staring at my grandmother. I was a super, super curious and victorious young person. I had to learn how to mask and refrain from being so creepy to others. There was another side, quiet and reserved, scared to take risks for fear of someone finding out I was not like the others. In the book, Living Independently on the Autism Spectrum, 2013. By: Lynne Soraya. Chapter 1, Skills for Self Advocacy ( pg. 26)

**"One way many people on the spectrum learn what to expect from others is to read about human behavior"**

Reading to understand the world around me became more than a passtime. Masking my way through. I had an entire set of neurotypical communication styles available to me just by observation. I could practice my skill and learn all in the same place. People watching became an obsession. I wasn't being included in much so people became my passtime.

This aided me in finding a middle ground, but what we don't build on a solid foundation will crumble. The thinking styles of different people became my obsession. Finding out why they choose to do the things that they do. How we as a people can make generational change. I wondered why I had to be made like this. There are loads of people who have strengths that are opposite mine. We would have complemented each other but they'd rather build a false narrative instead. Makes me sick.

On page 65, of Living Independently of the Autism Spectrum, By: Lynne Soraya. There are two points I'd like to point out.

- You can help others to understand you by using, "I tend to be…. Or " I'm the kind of person who…" Statements to communicate your differences and needs.

- One very important skill for being successful is learning to value and understand different communication and thinking styles of others.

Instead of masking and hiding ourselves, teach people how to treat you if you feel that the relationship is worth it. Let your boundaries and vulnerability be your guide. Muster up the courage to be authentically you.

# I'M TIRED OF WOMEN

## By: MissNatasha

Tired of women laughing at one another

Tired of women fighting one another

Tired of Fake women

Tired of pretentious women

Tired of manipulative women

Tired of women who don't care and lie like they do

Tired of women who don't tell you the real truth

Tired of gatekeeping women

Tired of women who think they're too much

Tired of women who are unsupportive

Tired of women who don't have faith

Tired of women who say they are one thing and do another

Tired of the women

Tired of women not owning up to their mistakes

Tired of women who say they care but have a funny way

of showing it

Tired of women who don't support one another

Tired of women who think there too good to apologize

Tired of women who don't have respect

Tired of women who can't be respectful

Tired of women who talk too much and don't know what they are talking about

Tired of women who didn't do their own work!

Tired of women without consideration

Tired of women who steal

Tired of women who steal others time; soul, spirit

Tired of women who don't love themselves!

Tired of women who don't know how to behave

Tired of women can't be trusted

Tired of women who can't be trusted with important jobs

Soo, tired of women who don't appreciate an autistic women like me but take my ideas; my style, my love, words, my care, my thoughts, misconstrue them and abuse them.

# MAY YOU ALWAYS BE GENTLE ON YOURSELF

-MissNatasha

# CHAPTER 6

# I FEEL LIKE ME, THE ME I SHOULD HAVE BEEN ALL ALONG

You're not welcome in our club. You aren't like us. Grade school highschool all over again, but wait we are in 2023.

Being neurodiverse isn't a walk in the park, believe me when I say I'm not fine with struggling and scrounging. Being taken advantage of can take a toll on a person no matter their ability. The only way to change these types of experiences is to have goals and save at least 10% of every dollar you earn. Being autistic is no excuse for not being prepared. Finding my place in the world is still a journey worth fighting for. No one was going to stop me from becoming great and providing for my family. What I didn't understand was that I WAS STOPPING ME. Then life came along and slapped me silly. I slipped and slid into a life that I didn't recognize designing. So I had to re-evaluate my priorities and goals. Pray and ask for forgiveness, mend wounds that were caused by me and forgive ones that were caused by others.

Using storytelling as a tool for healing; can be a positive space for immense transformative change. Ever since I was a child I would use stories as a way to escape tramas, big or small. I would make up stories and know in my heart that one day people all over the world would read them. I just needed to get out of my own way. I needed to take deep, deep inventory of my surroundings. And know that I am imperfectly and perfectly made. Allowing my God to do the rest.

Then start anew. This task was extremely difficult for me. The process made me lose a lot of pride and gain faith. I started to see people for who they truly were which at times was very hard to swallow let alone stomach. But here I am, a true authentic version of myself. Wearing my autism authentically. I am fully aware of what having autism has done for my life. Autism has shown me how to take life with a grain of salt. Take it or leave it. Love me or leave me this is who I was supposed to be. Forever evolving and striving for imperfection.

Be a good girl, Be nice. I was nice, I let others talk to me however they liked. I let people I didn't like force their whims upon me my choice wasn't an option. I felt like this about 70 to 80% of the time. The problem being so gullible. Clearly I took being the good girl too far. I didn't know any better, I didn't understand. I was a late bloomer. In my own world of fairy-tales and la la land. Don't show your frustration give others permish to violate multiple times. And let's not forget to smile. Stand straight and hide my own needs.

There were loads of times when I acted out. No one helped me to understand. Something had to give! I didn't believe that I could voice my thoughts and feelings to anyone. When I said no or expressed that I didn't like or did not want to participate, my prompts would be ignored. I started to mute myself. I learned to disconnect from my own wants and needs. My own emotions, To appease others. I know, I know it's not such a good thing to do. I grew to have a hyper vigilance for being the good girl. I was stuck in a state of avoiding conflict, indulging in service and avoiding my own thoughts and opinions. Without finding out who I was and why I'm here first. Again, I know, I know it's a bad idea. But I didn't see it at the time. Voicing what was on my mind came out in extremely discombobulated forms. Trying to assist others with their issues instead of fixing my situation should have been the first on the to do list. I was heavily in my feelings like I couldn't make a difference in life and I would always be here in this exact place. Was there something wrong with me? I started to question myself. Breaking this idea I had built in my head wasn't easy. There wasn't anything wrong, I just thought differently. And that's okay. The mere thought of some of you believing and living in the fullness of who you are just give me chills. Ooooh, the mere thought of what living authentically me would feel like; taste like. I'd bask in how blessed I would be. I would be at the helm of my own ship, not anyone else. Your authenticity is what makes you unique. That's what makes you awesome.

# BEE 🐝
## By: MissNatasha

BEE 🐝

BEE 🐝 Wise

BEE 🐝 GraceFilled

BEE 🐝 Genuine

BEE 🐝 Ambitious

BEE 🐝 Goal oriented

BEE 🐝 Forgiving

BEE 🐝 Careful

BEE 🐝 Ready

BEE 🐝 Fantastic

BEE 🐝 Persistent

BEE 🐝 Free

BEE 🐝 Healthy

BEE 🐝 Clean

BEE 🐝 New

BEE 🐝 Happy

BEE 🐝 Faithful

BEE 🐝 Diligent

BEE 🐝 Consistent

BEE 🐝 Special

BEE 🐝 Self sufficient

BEE 🐝 Kind

BEE 🐝 Stupendous

BEE 🐝 Thoughtful

BEE 🐝 Courageous

BEE 🐝 Prepared

BEE 🐝 Realistic

BEE 🐝 Confident

BEE 🐝 Honest

BEE 🐝 Pleasant

BEE 🐝 Well

BEE 🐝 GraceFilled

BEE 🐝 Genuine

BEE 🐝 You

BEE 🐝 Ambitious

BEE 🐝 Goal oriented

BEE 🐝 Forgiving

BEE 🐝 In control of your thoughts

**IT'S NOT BRAVERY**
**IF YOU DON'T FEEL FEAR, RIGHT?**
**IF YOUR NOT AFRAID,**
**THEN YOUR NOT REALLY**
**FORCING YOURSELF TO**
**DO SOMETHING BRAVE**

-Lisa Braswell

# CHAPTER 7
# JUST BREATHE

I was first introduced to parenting as a young person. I would watch my younger siblings and cousins. My second introduction to parenting was as a teen mom, the usual for someone like me. Young black and gullible as hell. I didn't express myself much. I'd use clothes to define my mood. I would stick out like a sore thumb. I felt like I brought the problems I faced on myself. I would beat myself up about it and propel my soul into a depressive state. Eager to make friends in my neighborhood, I made friends with the wrong crowd and found myself drugged, used and confused. This experience made me very angry and distant. Being the eldest made this news a grave disappointment to my family. I learned the act of "concealing not feeling" shout out to all you Frozen fans that understand the notion of Masking. Building a wall with all sorts of devices to keep others out. Sometimes even yourself. I recall being fearful of how I would take care of this little individual and what would become of us in the future. I did everything that the book I was given in teen mom class said. Try to stay calm; no alcohol, cigarettes, plenty of fruits and veggies. I wondered if I was worthy to bring up the child growing inside me. I didn't want to be a bum. I had specific aspirations as a mom. Like new moms I was nervous, inexperienced and alone. As he grew inside my tummy I played calming music and did my darndest to be calm and content. Medical care was important to me but I didn't want to be judged. I was taken advantage of by a boy down the street and his friends. My family broke, I was without a place to live, I had a child to feed. I found myself depressed, blamed, alone, fear filled and isolated. No way out. Going to get checked out was very humiliating and degrading but I still carried on.

For years I was treated and looked at like a zoo animal. I am just me, I can't help that I haven't made proper friendships; found a career at 25, saved 3 to six months of expenses or built boundaries.

I started going to teen moms groups to learn more about adulting and negative thoughts that may come up. I remembered one time when my 4-5 month old wouldn't stop crying. I was so frustrated. I went in and out of the room with no victory. I too started to cry. I placed him in my room on the bed with lots of blankets and pillows surrounding him so that he didn't roll off the bed and fall. I walked out of the room for a couple of mins or so to take a couple breaths.

In an article I read recently about the Kintsuji method and the art of repair. A 400 + year old repair method. This method emphasizes the nooks and cracks. With the emphasized golden cracks, the item is much more valuable and unique. Life is all about perspective. It is said that the feeling of regret when something is wasted and replaced with the need to accept change. When we change for the better after bad things happen we make life more rare, confident, and beautiful. I was supposed to be perfect, go and do great things. When I had experienced tramas I broke, I broke into a million pieces. This book is my way of showing you all that you can put yourself back together. God is like the materials used to place a broken item back together. Powdered gold; silver, platinum, an even richer substance than anything you can think of.

That's when I learned about breathing through my pain. The pain of not being able to communicate what was happening to my body to any professional person.  Some say that all they need is love but actually we need oxygen to the brain to function. We need oxygen to the heart for our hearts to function. Even the blood in our bodies needs oxygen.

Taking the time to take intentional breaths not only keeps you alive it also assists in mental and physical regulation. Which in turn allows for you to utilize more brain space for important tasks instead of foolishness. If I discussed how I felt when I was overwhelmed, I was told to just don't worry and ignore those feelings.

When you do, the worst comes out in those around you because you're not valuing yourself or your needs and wants. As we all have heard we CAN NOT assist anyone if our own life vest or oxygen mask isn't on first. They all would fluff me off and say if fine, just go home and relax.

# ASK

## By: MissNatasha

Ask me who my circle is don't assume

Ask me about who trusts me and who I trust

Ask me about what you hear, don't assume

Ask me about my triumphs

Ask me why they violate

Ask me if I feel Canadian

Ask me if they just use me

Ask me if they are kosher

Ask them if they had ablest intentions

Ask me if I've done my part or not

Ask me if I've done everything that I can do

Ask me if I gave it the old college try

Ask

Ask them why they pretend

Ask me if it rains, does it pour

Ask them if they're full of love or just hate

Ask them, Ask them if they're satisfied with their lives

Ask them if they're tired of gatekeeping

Ask them if they're happy

Ask them if they are running on E!

Ask them if they need a redo

Ask them if they need to say I'm sorry

Ask them if they're for filled

Ask them if they're joyous

Ask them if they're Grace filled

Ask them if they're lonely

Ask them if they really need a friend

Ask them if they self reflect

Ask them if they own up to their mistakes

Ask them if they're honest about trouble, they started

Ask them about their ego

Ask me before you assume

# CHAPTER 8: ACTION STEP #1

# LISTEN TO THE INNER VOICE INSIDE, YOUR FIRST MIND!

Listen to your first mind. You may be wondering what I mean by your first mind. Well, it's like your conscience, or your intuition , the little angel on your shoulder that helps you distinguish right from wrong. It's highly recommended that you pay close attention to this voice, because it will guide you to a deeper understanding of self. A deeper understanding of oneself results in a skilled and accomplished future. Having a deeper understanding of myself has also improved my understanding of others.

Throughout this process of trusting my first mind I stumbled hard and on top of the many, many times. I believe that it was due to the receptors in my brain. Or lack thereof. I felt as though I was not human. Feels of:

- Second guessing

- Doubting oneself and one's abilities

- Unbelief

- Lack of courage

- Low Self esteem

- Fear

Examples like this plagued my existence. I wore these feelings like one would wear those itchy stockings every week to church. We'd have to sit still and stand up, sing and smile on que or else you would hear whispers of whose grandchild is that? I learned to conform and conformity is the exact opposite to freedom. I was a glorified robot. Doing and acting in exactly the way I was programmed.

Deprogrammed

Not on my own terms

Unnatural

Forced

Pressure

Forced to swallow a heavy dose of reality, made me realize how much my brain didn't work like other people. When pressured I'd give in to the most unnatural of things. I thought that relationships were transactional. I believed that friendships were one sided. I felt pressured to fit into the square box. A time that stands out to me was when I worked as a Preschool readiness instructor, there was a time when a mom approached me in her mother tongue inquiring about her child being transferred to my classroom. I had to really dig deep to gather what this mother was trying to convey. I took deep breaths and focused my mind on the mom's eyes; mouth and hands. My observations led me to believe that this was a mother desperate for change. From what I gathered this mom wanted her child to be placed in my classroom because the other facilitator wasn't treating her child very well. This type of situation was not the first, this was the first of many.

I believe because I'm a woman; because I'm of a brown complexion, because of my unseen disabilities, I'm perceived as a liability more than an asset. What others don't seem to realize is that I have treasures that surpasses monetary value. When I was young I felt like a black sheep. I was out spoken, bold and wanted to be included in everything. I had a lot to ask and find out about the world.

As a mother we will go to any extent to provide the proper care for our children. I asked for the child's information and gestured to the front office for the mother to transfer her child to my classroom. A smile of relief came upon her face. I started to take walks in my down time at work. Listening to the birds and nature around me. I chose to pray and sing out my woes. Find deep, deep forgiveness for the place and people that I worked for. Building parent connections and guiding children into a big school one child at a time. Deprogramming my mind from the thought that the way I am conducting myself within my work space was every bit relevant. And what I was doing was important. If not the classroom wouldn't be full each and every quarter.

My breathing techniques and focused mind literally helped a mother and child that day. I would go outside for walks to breath and clear my mind for the next session of children, but that day was special. Start regulating your nervous system by breathing with intention, especially in high-stress situations. Be clear and focused on one problem at a time. You'll be able to make proper decisions for yourself, aligning with your true self if you take these action steps seriously. Take time to be quiet and listen to your body. Be still and know that you have the power within.

My conscience was my guide. Sometimes I would listen and other times I'd think I'm too good to listen. I would get knocks or taps on my shoulder, trying to tell me what to do. I asked around about it and most said that they didn't really listen to that voice. They'd shrug their shoulders and ignore the call. The thing is once ignored you can't come crying and whining about the repercussions. I'd cry and whine all the time. This is what is called stubbornness. My little gut feeling served me well. It was my curiosity that made me think twice. I had watched others take risks on television. Not taking into account that it was television. I'd use some of the lines I'd heard but it would always get me into trouble. I'd believe if I pleased others with their desires or needs that I'd eventually get what I needed from them as well. That there is what's called a conditional relationship. The only problem is I'd give most of myself in one way or another and not get what I needed in return. I'd get a version of what the other person thought I needed and I would be resentful and bitter about what I was receiving. Most times it was because I second guessed that little voice, telling me what I should think about instead of the other thing over there enticing me to do the wrong thing. This made life take longer. Learning lessons took longer. I believe it's a combination of listening to too many different opinions; not feeling like I belonged, stubbornness and lack of confidence.  I didn't see myself reflected in anyone around me which left me feeling disconnected, discombobulated. I looked to fictional characters and sports professionals, tv characters for comfort and strength. The maneuvers that these characters fictional or real life had the skills and know how to get the job done and I was determined to do the same.

# TOO MUCH

## BY: MISSNATASHA

I've been in too many rooms

Too loud; too colourful, too energetic, too ADHD, too sad, too MAD, too fearful, too cheerful, too empathetic, too Autistic, too spiritual, too deep, too sexy, too inquisitive, too CPTSD, too shameful, too prideful, too nice, too much spice, too patient, too frank, too peaceful, too flavourful , too respectful, too heavy, too energetic, too commercial, too 2001, too free, too negative, too smart for my own good, too creative, too extraordinary, too foreign, too bashment, too basic, too interested, too available, too compromised, too expensive, too comfortable, too dark, too light, too much freedom, too innocent, too sporty, too nerdy, too too religious, too superstitious, too small, too big, too suppressed, too compromised, too kind, too focused, too medicated, too naive, too dense, too stuck, too slow, too fast, too undecided, too put together, too much labels, too obsessed, too spacey, too ambiguous, too freaky, too argumentative, too foolish, too cheap, too fit, too compromised, too calm, to solid, too quiet, too funny, too powerful beyond measure, too complete, too street, too late, too frequent, too quarky, too suburban, too black, too white, too frustrated, too comfortable, too

wobbly, too sensitive, too turvy, too plain, too special,
too creative, too knowledgeable, too modern, too old
school, too jumpy, too involved, too me, too dismissive,
too inclusive, too Autistic, too obvious, too spontaneous,
too caring, too sweet, too much silence, too sour, too
polished, too eloquent, too enthusiastic, too messy,
too tidy, too simple, too grounded, too out there, too
consuming , too forced, too forceful, too painful, too
risky! Too extreme, too long, too skilled, too scared, too
needy, too loving, too bright, too far, too direct, too
vague, too heavy, too silent, too general, too open, too
closed, too important, too preferred, too sudden, too
typical, too privileged, too entitled, too connected, too
removed, too belted, too over sexualized, too emotional,
too graceful, too dramatic, too forward, too soulful,
too serious, too proactive,  too magical, too motivated,
too consistent, too commercial, too whitewashed, too
fortunate, too unfortunate, too needy, too tired, too
friendly, too nice, too busy, too gross, too squeamish,
too current, too touchy, too sunny, too capable, too
attached, too relevant, too influential, too mindful,
too sincere, too submissive, to warm, too cold, too
afraid, too senile, too weak, too tired, too degrading,
too fantastical, too sorry, too you, too supportive,
too worthy, too connected, too prioritized, too bad,
too much further, too accessible, too segregated, too
accustomed, too behaved, too well mannered, too
unruly, too privileged, too fabulous, too consumed, too
compassionate, too perfect, too valued, too still, too
honest, too many assumptions, too fantastical, too good
for you, too much garbage, too developed, too many
mistakes, too frequent, too significant, too truthful, too
separated, too mean, too calm, too isolated, too out of
control, too controlling, too accusatory, too fascinating,

too general, too extreme, too conflicting, too accepting, too in control, too offended, too misunderstood, too different, too reactive, too unstoppable, too calculated, too cruel, too experienced, too balanced, too risky, too fascinating, too genuine, too clueless, too used, too content, too fowl, too unhealthy, too much people pleasing, too much distractions, too much self doubt, too much negative thoughts, too much, too forthcoming, too much to stomach, too deliberate, too much procrastination, too annoying, too withholding, too technical, too valid, too extra, too romantic, too much perspective, too credible, too committed, too dangerous, too prideful, too much problems, too much fury, too segmented, too dysfunctional, too tenderhearted, too insecure, too harsh, too satisfied, too comfortable, too many decisions, too important, too much encouragement, too many grudges, too settled, too tremendous, too many victims, too many betrayals, too much crying, too much pain, too set in their ways, too polite, too gentle, too fascinating, too distant, too much vigour, too disconnected, too disabled, too mysterious, too moral, too ethical, too many patterns, Too Blessed to be stressed

# CHAPTER 9: ACTION STEP #2

# MAKE DECISIONS THAT ALIGN WITH YOUR VALUES AND BELIEF SYSTEMS.

Know what you value! For instance I value being with authentically awesome people that care and value me and others. It was a pattern of mine to be around people who didn't really value me because I didn't value myself enough. I let low level individuals talk down to me. I thought that it was disobedient to speak up. I am not going to continue to be around individuals that my mind and body don't agree with. As a youth I would have hazard signs on certain individuals. What do I mean by hazard signs? People that my body and mind are telling me something is wrong and I don't listen. I would consistently give any opinions for individuals to disrespect and devalue me as a human. I became disgruntled. Because I valued others before myself this gave free reign for others to stomp on me. Having values and morals is crucial to a well balanced life. I had to Google generic values and find a few that I resonated with to build the proper life that I deserved. You can definitely find at least five or ten values that speak to you, these values will serve as your rules and regulations for life moving forward. Your values will be weighed; poked and tested but stay the course! Although some of my values started to form as a child. I began to compile my values even more while attending Teen mom group. And as I got older I started to see the errors of my ways and pivot to new more longer lasting values and beliefs. Like, giving thanks when I wake and spending time with my creator. Do the inner work to focus on upholding your values.

Through watching my grandmother volunteer and give back informed me that giving back is a part of living a healthy life. Volunteering within the teen mom group. My grandmothers taught me that acts of service are 100% one of my values.

Feel free to redo and reconstruct your values if needed. I decided one of the major values in my life would be to significantly reduce my masking. Masking for me was like trying to fit into a pea sized bead. I tried to mold myself into what wasn't for me. Like I'm not going to go to a horror show if I'm deathly afraid of horror movies. I'll support a friend in a different manner. The thought of masking just to please others has me thinking twice.  I believed that being authentically myself was too much or not enough, I was way too hard on myself, plus it was becoming exhausting. Masking can hurt the nervous system. Be aware of the situations you put yourself into as much as possible. I didn't really grasp the severity of some of the situations I put myself in until it was too late. The receptors in my brain weren't connecting I guess. Some would say I have a tough head. That was only a part of the problem. I believed in others before I had faith and belief in myself. I actually will renege that statement and say that I stopped believing in myself as a young teen.

# COLLABORATION OVER COMPETITION

# CHAPTER 10: ACTION STEP #3

## SETTING BOUNDARIES AND WALKING AWAY FROM TOXIC SITUATIONS.

In my case, after I started to find my voice and call out certain movements that I knew were wrong. Family and friends started to dissipate.Once I started to assert myself and fluff up my feathers with confidence. I asked God to see how others looked at me, I asked for wisdom and grace to see things clearly. Wow, let me tell you that when you ask the Lord for wisdom. Mercy, your life and everything in it will reveal what is happening around you. Inevitably by implementing boundaries and walking away from toxic situations will result in losing a lot of people who benefited from you being docile and unaware. It was strange to me because I didn't have anything really to give but I found that others would take the weirdest things. My style or a phrase. A funny joke or a suggestion.  As an autistic adult I know now how much boundaries are absolutely vital in one's life NOW. I beat myself up about it a lot. But either IceT or Ice Cube said. "Don't cry over the work that you didn't put in." It's a hard but cold fact!

Being Neurodivergent has come with soooo many assumptions. An interesting internal monologue,

*Assumptions kill! I think that I am unable to do anything. My imagination is very robust , vivid and I don't know what reality is. I don't know what the intentions are of others but in actuality the senses are heightened.*

I'm a fairly intelligent person and hearing those same old assumptions the majority of the time from family and friends can take a toll on you. If you want to know something ask! If you're curious about why I don't go to gatherings anymore, ask! I noticed if you're in disruptive situations or family dynamics that aren't suiting the person you are growing out of. Stop talking to the people around you about your plans. Those who mean you no good will take your temperature for others. Ask if there is anything they can do, in order to prolong their stay in your life. They will blame you often and reluctantly want to resolve or see their part in the problem. Effort in a family or friendship looks like. Communicating to resolve not to blame. I have a family who refuse to see me in a positive light and there is nothing on this GOD's GREEN Earth that caused it but the fact that I touch insecurities in them. Not because of my wrong doings. In fact when confronted they hardened and doubled down. I absolutely don't need to involve myself with individuals or high control groups formed specifically for someone else's controlled pleasure. Thank GOD almighty that we are differently and wonderfully made and HE taught and is teaching me how to truly love and care for others no matter if they deserve it or not. All of that: ***Ghosting and Roasting; Blaming and Gaming, Score Keeping and Holy than thou antics are Played Out!*** We are all going to have to come correct for the things that we've done sooner or later. I am not going to be bullied into being around people who don't care about me and my family. That's why when starting a family you must have boundaries with your family members and know what both will and will not tolerate within that family. Kept my family too up close and personal into the affairs of my life. And when I didn't want them involved because they were not healthy, many ignored violations later. Some will do sneaky, sneaky underhanded things to be involved and then say that it's not them it was the one eyed man. Either way the fact is now there has to be a clear indication as to why we stopped talking in order to start healthy communication. Someone said somewhere: Silence isn't an apology! I never got it back then. They'd violate and go Silent and then pop up again and again. I asked for guidance on this matter from the man upstairs and HE worked it out for me. Well it worked itself out. I was an easy target and I'm a big suck too. I learned my lessons and have clearly found that We must lean not on our own understandings. Setting boundaries comes with complaints; change, and connection to self. One form of toxicity can come in the form of  negative people that you associate with. You don't wanna be a part of a peer group that only talks or gossips about others or a peer group that doesn't ever move forward. This type of situation may be easy to decipher for some. But for me I second guessed myself alot and other people around me would capitalize on it. I don't have much to offer so I wondered what is it about me? Some of us would stay in degrading, damaging situations because we don't believe that we can find proper encouraging uplifting relationships.We have to have the love and self confidence to leave relationships that do not serve us. Being aware of what your toxic traits are and how those traits can be triggered is an effective way to combat toxicity. Combating negative thoughts, actions from others. You know those negative types of people! Or situations that tend to blame the person with the disability before the ignorance of organizational politics.

You know those three or four trips to the fast food restaurant will do to you! You know of that one coworker that continues to be a downer each and everyday! You have no business fraternizing with these types of toxic traits because you are on another level now! Being able to decrease the stressors in your life.

In Nedra Glover Tawwab's book, Set Boundaries find peace she gives some examples of boundaries and why we need them. Here are just a few:

- **Boundaries define roles in relationships**

- **Boundaries are ways to create healthy relationships**

- **Boundaries communicate acceptable and unacceptable behaviors in relationships**

- **Boundaries are a way to feel safe**

As a young woman, I didn't not implement boundaries. And I went along with what was said, regardless if I felt it was right or not. I had not built values and systems that would have helped me manage my life more effectively. I knew that I was a mother but if another mom came around and criticized what I was doing I'd feel bad about my own parenting and change. Listening when they'd say I'm too young or too slow. Stuffies help me be at peace, so do books, and writing. Not having very much belief in myself when it came to certain tasks. Mainly came from the people I was around. I started to notice patterns and attitudes, behaviors and lack of accountability, in both myself and others.

The wings of change are coming. I wouldn't let others know when they violated me, keeping the feelings to myself. Acting out when I couldn't cope and isolated until I was over it. I would keep myself in spaces where no one would get me. I was misunderstood. I was like a mascot or pet. I didn't like the feeling but it was better than being by myself . I soon learned that being alone was better than squeezing to fit in a circle when you're a star.

# SOME PEOPLE DON'T RATE THE TORTOISE BUT THE TORTOISE GETS THE JOB DONE!

## -MissNatasha 2020

# WATER YOUR PLANS!

Water your plans, what do I mean by this? You are a gem, a wonderful you. Take time to implement. Implement your voice when necessary. Your voice is important to your happiness. Know when to take initiative within your own life. Taking breaks without explanation, embracing rejection, and not taking rejection personally. I embrace failure to win. Watering your plans means building a plan of your own goals and aspirations. Finding positive and worthwhile dreams to achieve. What does that look like? Look at who you have around you. How do they make you feel? Taking inventory doesn't have to be reported to anyone. This process is for you to become aware of who you are surrounding yourself with.

# FAITH IT
## UNTIL YOU MAKE IT
## AND HAVE THE
## GODFIDENCE TO
## SEE THINGS THROUGH
### -MissNatasha

# CONCLUSION

As I conclude, This book will pose self reflection opportunities.. Providing points on how one can overcome the negative nancy's: trials, tribulations, those violin songs.

I know that not understanding who I was from a younger age played a part in my journey. I had courage but it was misguided and reckless. I would be undercover happy. Drinking and partying my Tramas away. When someone would suggest I do something like go out to celebrate. I would say yes even though I knew I should have said no. Heavily wanting to fit in. I would use the victim excuse to prove to myself that I needed to go out and treat myself. This cycle did nothing for me. Made me, Blue. Blue started to emerge in late highschool.

Blue was bold and rude. Never really caring about much of anything. Blue would dress provocatively and party. Blue had no backbone and didn't know how to build boundaries. Blue didn't know how to deal with big tramas. A disaster. A shit show! Unable to say no and a doormat. I wanted to be normal so bad that I compromised everything. Conformity is the worst! I didn't know that my disabilities were my gifts, and I possessed my own freedom with God and faith. My Abilities will come and I could share them with the world. It was a very devastating time in my life. With disabilities you can be bamboozled into thinking that they are not normal but what is normal?

When I was growing up, I had to ask questions over and over again about tasks my parents asked of me. Too many questions. I couldn't help it. I got the gist that I was annoying; repetitive,  and because I am very blunt it was seen as rude. I was disgruntled about not being understood everywhere I went. I heard it plenty from family.I didn't really have friends. Made me low key disheartened. There were times my attention would wander or my interest in something would fade or increase. This must have been very troublesome to my family. My interests would deepen tremendously depending on the certain topics. I had fixated on various topics over the years. Teaching; Counseling, Animals, Sex, the body, pop culture.

Observing how others did things would be an obsession of mine. I would help when asked and as I got older I would be so fixated on a subject or something I'm doing I'd have to be pulled away. My parents showed me how to maneuver myself within this Canadian world. Cold; hot, hot, cold. Canadian weather is very unpredictable. And as I said earlier I ask a lot of questions and make loads of observations.  My parents came to Canada to build a life outside of Grenada and Jamaica. I was the first born, one cold snowy February.

Playing kick ball barefoot wasn't my story and it took some trips and storytelling to overstand the reasoning behind what my parents were trying to teach me.  I appreciated overhearing stories of Jamaica and Grenada. I wanted to know all about how my parents maneuvered themselves back home. How they maneuvered themselves here in Canada. I wished I could have heard more about life in the west indies. I love my parents dearly for believing in themselves enough to do something big, for a bigger purpose. I must say my parents are strong and purposeful people! Dedicated and hardworking individuals. I didn't really understand all of what they were sharing with me at the time but I can honestly say that it has become very apparent the older I got.

Why do our parents stress the particular areas they stress? I believe our parents have a duty to share what they've been taught from their parents. I wanted to know if my parents knew if I was different. When did they realize? Being able to sustain my own family without anyone's help, that was is and forever will be my goal. I dreamed of being like everyone else. But in actuality I am nothing close to normal! Unusual; peculiar, different. Those for sure. I dreamt of calm and a white picket fence; music a blare while I prepare for supper. My children coming home to enjoy dinner at home. Sustaining myself and my family. Transfer the Lord's teachings to my own children. Transferring what I've been taught from my  parents and grandparents. I remember loads because of my parents and grandparents, I have a blueprint for greatness. The neurons connect differently. I gotta be gentle with my brain. I believe I got side tracked and started using bad traits without even strategically thinking.

This happens when you don't plan. Life makes plans for you. Disabilities or not. Now it's up to me to build on what was started. You are supposed to use your gifts for good and the enrichment of others. I have a saying " You can only be you, that's all you can do" So do you! Do you with intention and authority,

Do you with gusto and grit, Do you with Exceptional Excellence!

I received honors in university because of advocating for myself. Speaking up for myself, assisting others to find their own voices. During my 20 years in preschool readiness I provided opportunities for learning through play. By being kind; open to diversity, learning styles and differences. For each and every child that I interacted with.

The excuse of the child being troublesome or difficult is not flying anymore! You will find resilience, strength, and hope in each and everyone of us no matter the diagnosis or color. Of Course use your discretion and intuition when interacting with anyone. Do you as best as you possibly can!

Reading this book should inspire you to check yourself and reflect on yourself! You'll learn something new or even share some knowledge learned. I hope this book assists you in finding the most authentic parts of yourself so you can share your strengths and creativity with the world. This world needs people willing to do the work to be great, then share those gifts with the world. How do you navigate hope? Remember you can only be you, that's all you can do! Turning the pages of this book, issues of how learning in a Canadian classroom was like growing up; how I crushed self doubt, and ventured off into the land of self love and acceptance, How I built boundaries for myself and others, built solutions to changing issues internal and external. The subject of inner transformation and loving the human you were born to be regardless of diagnosis or another's opinion.

# SHARE YOUR SUNSHINE
## BY: MISSNATASHA

Share your Sunshine  with the world

Share your Sunshine  with a smile

Share your Sunshine  with a song

Share your Sunshine  with your voice

Share your Sunshine  with your creativity

Share your Sunshine  a kind word

Share your Sunshine  by doing good

Share your Sunshine  by standing out

Share your Sunshine  by doing the right thing

Share your Sunshine  by being kind

Share your Sunshine  sharing a story with a friend

Share your Sunshine  with the people around you

Share your Sunshine  by being brave

Share your Sunshine  by speaking up

Share your Sunshine  by using your intuition

Share your Sunshine with strangers

Share your Sunshine everyday

Share your Sunshine with others

Share your Sunshine and be true to you

**Let's build Connection and Community with NatashaConnects**

**LinkTree:**
https://linktr.ee/NatashaConnects

Check out - The **CreateDon'tHate** show on YouTube

# -AFRICAN PROVERB-

**The African Consciousness Bookstore says:
An educator in a system of oppression is either a revolutionary or
an oppressor**

# WHICH ONE ARE YOU???

CREATE DON'T HATE

**BROKEN THINGS CAN BECOME BLESSED THINGS IF YOU LET GOD DO THE MENDING**

## REFERENCES:

Sept 19, 2019, Andrea Mantovani KINTSUGI AND THE ART OF REPAIR: life is what makes us
https://medium.com/@andreamantovani/kintsugi-and-the-art-of-repair-life-is-what-makes-us-b4af13a3992

Movie: Come as You Are; a 2019

Documentary - Autism in Love 2015 - PBS special

The Golden Compass: by Philip Pullman, 31 July 2019
https://www.litcharts.com/lit/the-golden-compass/symbols/the-alethiometer

Song: Bag Lady, Released: 2000, Album: Mama's Gun, Artist: Erykah Badu

Sexual Knowledge, Desires, and Experience of Adolescents and Young Adults With an Autism Spectrum Disorder: An Exploratory Study
Crossref DOI link: https://doi.org/10.3389/fpsyt.2021.685256
Published Online: 2021-06-09

https://www.ncbi.nlm.nih.gov/pmc/articles/PMC5572253/
Huang AX, Hughes TL, Sutton LR, Lawrence M, Chen X, Ji Z, Zeleke W. Understanding the Self in

Individuals with Autism Spectrum Disorders (ASD): A Review of Literature. Front Psychol. 2017 Aug 22;8:1422. doi: 10.3389/fpsyg.2017.01422. PMID: 28878717; PMCID: PMC5572253.
https://www.independent.co.uk/news/uk/home-news/adults-with-learning-disabilities-at-risk-of-abuse-say-charities-9909302.html

Lawson, W. B. (2020). Adaptive morphing and coping with social threat in autism: an autistic perspective. Journal of Intellectual Disability - Diagnosis and Treatment, 8(3), 519-526. https://doi.org/10.6000/2292-2598.2020.08.03.29

https://www.scarymommy.com/parenting-special-needs-always-on/
I'm A Mom Of A Child With Special Needs....And I'm So Tired
by Jenn Jones January 12, 2021 Updated February 19, 2021

https://www.nytimes.com/2015/05/03/opinion/sunday/what-black-moms-know.html
What Black Moms Know By Ylonda Gault Caviness May 2, 2015

https://www.scarymommy.com/moms-black-boys-special-needs-terrified-right-now/
Moms Of Black Boys With Special Needs Are Terrified
by Rachel Garlinghouse June 17, 2020

https://leanin.org/black-women-racism-discrimination-at-work#!
Lean in. org

# ABOUT THE AUTHOR

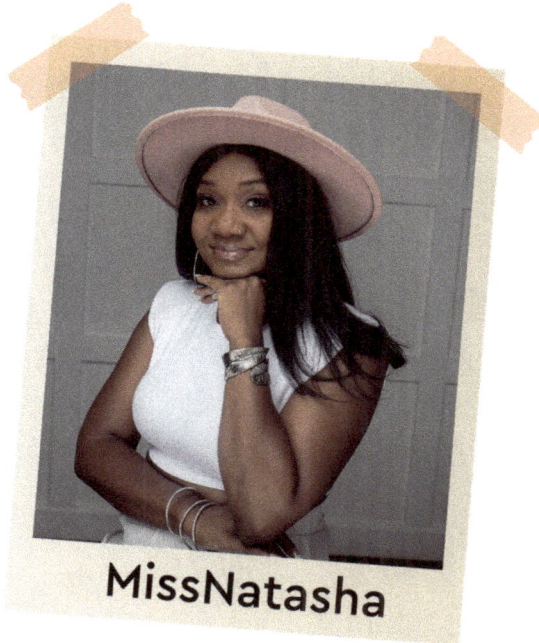

MissNatasha

Good Morning, Good Afternoon, Good Evening and Good Night everyone. MissNatasha here, I hope that you are doing well. MissNatasha is a Mental Wellness Creator and Disability Advocate; Speaker and Author. MissNatasha is a mother of two and auntie to many. MissNatasha resides in Toronto, Canada, and is Authentically Autistic /ADHD, among other wonderful things. MissNatasha is the creator of Create Don't Hate, a show on YouTube. MissNatasha's intention is that you will leave the pages of this story with a greater appreciation of one person's Neurodivergent experience. Look inward for the goodness inside you.

YOU CAN ONLY **BE YOU,** THAT'S ALL YOU **CAN DO!**

-MissNatasha

www.ingramcontent.com/pod-product-compliance
Lightning Source LLC
Chambersburg PA
CBHW051259020426
42333CB00026B/3272